# Endurance Sport and the American Philosophical Tradition

# American Philosophy Series

*Series Editor:* John J. Kaag, University of Massachusetts Lowell

*Advisory Board:* Charlene Haddock Siegfried, Joe Margolis, Marilyn Fischer, Scott Pratt, Douglas Anderson, Erin McKenna, and Mark Johnson

The *American Philosophy Series* at Lexington Books features cutting-edge scholarship in the burgeoning field of American philosophy. Some of the volumes in this series are historically oriented and seek to reframe the American canon's primary figures: James, Peirce, Dewey, and DuBois, among others. But the intellectual history done in this series also aims to reclaim and discover figures (particularly women and minorities) who worked on the outskirts of the American philosophical tradition. Other volumes in this series address contemporary issues—cultural, political, psychological, educational—using the resources of classical American pragmatism and neo-pragmatism. Still others engage in the most current conceptual debates in philosophy, explaining how American philosophy can still make meaningful interventions in contemporary epistemology, metaphysics, and ethical theory.

### Recent titles in the series

*Endurance Sport and the American Philosophical Tradition*, by Douglas R. Hochstetler
*Reconstructing the Personal Library of William James: Markings and Marginalia from the Harvard Library Collection* by Ermine L. Algaier IV
*Pragmatist and American Philosophical Perspectives on Resilience* edited by Kelly A. Parker and Heather E. Keith
*Rorty, Religion, and Metaphysics* by John Owens
*Ontology after Philosophical Psychology: The Continuity of Consciousness in William James's Philosophy of Mind*, by Michela Bella
*The Pragmatism and Prejudice of Oliver Wendell Holmes, Jr.,* edited by Seth Vannatta
*Richard Rorty and the Problem of Postmodern Experience: A Reconstruction*, by Tobias Timm
*Peirce and Religion: Knowledge, Transformation, and the Reality of God*, by Roger A. Ward
*William James, Moral Philosophy, and the Ethical Life,* edited by Jacob L. Goodson
*Epistemic Issues in Pragmatic Perspective*, by Nicholas Rescher
*Loving Immigrants in America: An Experiential Philosophy of Personal Interaction*, by Daniel G. Campos
*The Religious Dimension of Experience: Gabriel Marcel and American Philosophy*, by David W. Rodick
*Aesthetic Transcendentalism in Emerson, Peirce, and Nineteenth-Century American Landscape Painting*, by Nicholas L. Guardiano

# Endurance Sport and the American Philosophical Tradition

Edited by
Douglas Hochstetler

Foreword by
Amby Burfoot

LEXINGTON BOOKS
*Lanham • Boulder • New York • London*

Published by Lexington Books
An imprint of The Rowman & Littlefield Publishing Group, Inc.
4501 Forbes Boulevard, Suite 200, Lanham, Maryland 20706
www.rowman.com

6 Tinworth Street, London SE11 5AL, United Kingdom

Copyright © 2020 The Rowman & Littlefield Publishing Group, Inc.

Excerpt from Scott Tinley 2016, email to author reprinted with permission from Scott Tinley.

Parts of Chapter 11 have appeared previously in the author's book, *Finding Triathlon* (Hatherleigh, 2015). Reprinted with permission.

Material from: Ron Welters, *Towards a Sustainable Philosophy of Endurance Sport*, 2019 Springer Nature Switzerland AG, reproduced with permission of SNCSC

*All rights reserved.* No part of this book may be reproduced in any form or by any electronic or mechanical means, including information storage and retrieval systems, without written permission from the publisher, except by a reviewer who may quote passages in a review.

British Library Cataloguing in Publication Information Available

The hardback edition of this book was previously catalogued by the Library of Congress as follows:

**Library of Congress Cataloging-in-Publication Data Available**

Library of Congress Control Number: 2019954145

ISBN: 978-1-4985-4781-9 (cloth)
ISBN: 978-1-4985-4783-3 (pbk.)
ISBN: 978-1-4985-4782-6 (electronic)

# Contents

Foreword   vii
*Amby Burfoot*

Acknowledgments   xi

Introduction: The Nature of American Philosophy
and Endurance Sport   xiii
*Douglas Hochstetler*

1   Running and Musing: Living Philosophically   1
    *Douglas Anderson*

2   When Continentalism Meets Pragmatism: Enduring
    Life in the Strenuous Mood   11
    *Ron Welters*

3   Floyd Landis, Endurance Sport and the Aesthetics of Tension   31
    *Tim Elcombe*

4   Sunrise, Sunset: Reflections on What Makes an
    Aging Biker's Life Significant   49
    *Scott Kretchmar*

5   Representative Endurance Athlete   61
    *Peter Hopsicker*

6   Cooking up a Plan: Pragmatism and Training   79
    *Pam R. Sailors and Cody D. Cash*

| | | |
|---|---|---|
| 7 | Dewey Goes the Distance: Situated Habit and Ultraendurance Sports<br>*Jesús Ilundáin-Agurruza, Shaun Gallagher, Daniel D. Hutto, and Kaarina Beam* | 97 |
| 8 | "The Will to Believe," the Will to Win, and the Problem of Self-Transcendence<br>*Jeffrey Fry* | 125 |
| 9 | On Meaning and Motive in Endurance Sport: An Experiential Romp through the Grand Whys<br>*Scott Tinley* | 143 |

Conclusion: Circles of Life: Evaluating Goals and Preparing for the Future — 159
*Douglas Hochstetler*

Index — 171

Contributor Biographies — 173

# Foreword

Recently, I saw one of those newspaper articles about the benefits of exercise, specifically running. The researchers presented reams of data to support their contention that running extends life. But they knew they would face skeptics. Some would sneer: "What good is an extra hour if you had to endure an hour of running to achieve it?"

So the researchers crunched their numbers, and reported that every hour of running actually produces seven hours of longer life. I immediately got out a pen and pad of paper. I wanted to figure out all the miles (and hours) I've spent on the run the last fifty-five years. I wasn't, however, trying to determine if I might become a centenarian.

No, I found a different question far more intriguing: How much time have I spent running and thinking? After all, I've never run with a radio, podcasts, iTunes, or audiobooks. I run, and I listen to myself. I listen to that unpredictable flow of thoughts that moving feet always seem to unleash.

I also wondered: What have I learned from all this running and thinking?

The first question, I can answer. I've filled roughly 16,000 hours with running. That's edging up toward two years.

The second question is tougher. What have I got to show for 16,000 hours of free-range thinking? I simply don't know. There's not a shred of tangible evidence that I have been productive on the run. In fact, I can't remember 99 percent of the thoughts I have had on the tracks, trails, and roads. They have come, they have gone, there is no record of their existence.

Yet, I don't regret a single hour of my running time, and I look forward to harboring new thoughts, however briefly, on my next workout. I run, therefore I think. I can't assign a high ROI to this time. Conversely, how do you value 60 minutes of quiet, uninterrupted contemplation in a Twitterverse? I rate it very highly indeed.

I was lucky to have great, natural-born philosophers as guru (teachers) when I was young. They encouraged me to think free. My high school coach, John J. Kelley, won the 1957 Boston Marathon and ran in two Olympic Marathons, but never spoke of these events. Instead, he read and reread Thoreau, and aimed to strip his own existence to the absolute essentials.

It wasn't easy in the Mad Men era of the 1950s. The country was hell bent on "progress," which generally meant making things bigger and more consumptive. Kelley was a marathoner, vegetarian, and organic gardener who rode a bicycle to his public school teaching job rather than relying on the "infernal combustion machine," as he called the beat-up family car.

At my first college cross-country practice in 1964, I met psychiatrist Charley Robbins, who would eventually run the Manchester (CT) Road Race on fifty consecutive Thanksgiving-Day mornings. Robbins wore torn khaki pants and a ratty wool sweater against the chill. And nothing on his feet. He joined us collegians, 20 years younger than he, for a quick six-miler. Barefoot.

Kelley and Robbins showed me, early on, that one could take Robert Frost's road "less traveled by," and turn it into a path to excellence. Moreover, success didn't require fancy trappings. You could get there with simple grit and infinite passion. I took readily to their lessons.

At Runner's World, I worked for nearly two decades with Dr. George Sheehan, and conducted the last formal interview with him before his death from prostate cancer in 1993. Sheehan inspired me and millions with his monthly RW column, full of competitive zeal and philosophical meanderings.

A champion runner at every distance from the mile to the marathon, Sheehan found a wide audience by declaring that every runner and every race represented individual expression. Speed didn't matter. Only braveness. "Success means having the courage, the determination, and the will to become the person you were meant to be," he wrote.

In recent years, I have been stunned, and then thrilled, by the newfound interest in the neurobiology of running. When I started running five-plus decades ago, no one cared about anything but cholesterol, $VO_2$ max, and cardiovascular health. Now we learn almost every day about research breakthroughs in the physiology of neuro-fitness.

In other words, a fit heart is closely connected to a fit brain. Doh! What took us so long?

I'm sure this connection comes as no surprise to the philosophy students reading this book. You must have suspected the link all along. Why else would the worlds of running and philosophy have such a large intersection?

It's all about oxygen flow to the brain. That's why we can't turn off the stream of consciousness when we run. The feet move first, the heart responds with greater pumping, and the brain has no choice but to keep pace.

## Foreword

This is precisely the reason I so look forward to my next run—for the thoughts I will encounter there. Without the run, they might never surface.

Amby Burfoot
Mystic, CT
2019

Amby Burfoot won the 1968 Boston Marathon, served as Runner's World editor in chief for nearly two decades, and finished the 2018 Boston Marathon on the 50th anniversary of his victory. He has run 110,000 lifetime miles, and his most recent book is titled *Run Forever*.

# Acknowledgments

As I wrote two chapters for this book, worked with the authors to edit their writing, and conceptualized the project, I reflected on my gratitude for many people who shared their support and insights with me along the way.

Dave Nonnemacher—my college resident director and friend. Dave introduced me to an organization called Wandering Wheels which led me to two consecutive summers spent riding bike across the United States with a group of 50+ other like-minded individuals.

Dave Ackerman—my running partner and friend for more than fifteen years. When my family moved to Pennsylvania, I joined Dave on weekend runs and eventually reidentified as a runner. Since that time, Dave and I have run countless miles together including the Harrisburg Marathon and many half-marathons.

Michael Drabenstott (our "Oval Office" group leader) and my Wednesday morning track workout buddies. We meet at 5:15 am each week year-round, supporting each other, encouraging one another.

Rich Lally—my teammate for the Tussey Mountainback 50-mile relay race, grad school classmate and, more importantly, friend. A former Ironman-distance competitor, Rich allowed me to join his Penn State triathlon course and helped me believe I could, one day, run a marathon.

Peter M. Hopsicker—my friend, Penn State colleague, and partner for the Runner's World Half-Marathon Festival each year. We spend the weekend pushing each other in the various races (5k and 10k on Saturday; half-marathon on Sunday), pursuits which give clarity to our coauthored papers.

R. Scott Kretchmar, Douglas Anderson—grad school professors and significant mentors in many ways. I learned from them in classes focused on sport philosophy. They both modeled the active life and invested deeply in their students—for these reasons I'm forever grateful.

The other contributors—I am thankful for their willingness to join this book project. Many of these individuals are valued friends and with whom I have had the opportunity to run in places such as State College, PA; Prague, Tokyo, London, Porto, and Edinburgh.

Marty Gingerich—my initial running inspiration. My first cousin, 3 years older than me and an eventual state cross-country champion, I saw his dedication to training and his ability to remain humble in spite of his accomplishments and talent.

Penn State University—I am thankful for a semester-long sabbatical and opportunity to focus on this project.

Jana Hodges-Kluck—for her steady and guiding publishing hand at Rowman & Littlefield Publishing, dedicated to helping me bring this collection of works to print.

Family—for Mom and Dad, who modeled an active life and supported me through many sport seasons; for my children (Conley, Emma, Cora, and Erick) who are gifted in so many ways and have all joined me on runs at some point; for my wife, Heidi, and her unfailing support of me over the past twenty-three years of our marriage—I am blessed beyond measure.

# Introduction

## *The Nature of American Philosophy and Endurance Sport*

Douglas Hochstetler

In his book *Writing from the Center*, Scott Sanders (1995) raises a question regarding meaning and the nature of centeredness, asking: "How can one live a meaningful, gathered life in a world that seems broken and scattered?" His answer to this question is as follows: "To be centered, as I understand it, means to have a home territory, to be attached in a web of relationships with other people, to value common experience, and to recognize that one's life rises constantly from inward depths" (Sanders, 1995, ix).

Like Sanders, I have a deeply personal sense that living with meaning, with intent, is crucial and yet incredibly difficult in the twenty-first century. My concern here is how endurance sport meshes with and, perhaps even enhances, a pursuit of and engagement with the "good life" or, put another way, a life of significance. This is a topic I pursue daily as I lace up my shoes and head out the door to run. Anderson and Lally (2004), too, have this mindset. "Our own primary motive," they write, "seems to be that endurance training provides the setting for a sustained inquiry into the meaning and import of our own lives, to the lessons of suffering and possibility, as well as of failure and loss" (17).

In the context of both my personal and professional life, I have wrestled with these essential issues. In the context of this book, the questions remain. As such, to what extent, and in what ways, does endurance sport play at least a small part in our quest to live a meaningful and gathered life in a world that is so harried? Furthermore, how does a daily ritual, or to use MacIntyre's (1984) term, a practice, like running coexist with other commitments such as work and family? In this first chapter, my aim is to set the ground work for the chapters to follow. In the process I explore the nature of the American philosophical tradition, the nature of endurance sport, how this sport practice community intersects with American philosophy, and the extent to which a regional philosophical tradition has a potential bearing on both endurance sport and American philosophy.

Within the American philosophical tradition, Henry David Thoreau provides at least one example of a life pointed toward answering these questions regarding meaning—both personally and in the context of society. His time spent living at Walden Pond, two years of relative solitude apart from societal life, represents an experiment with intentional living, a portion of time dedicated toward his "personal business" of reading, writing, and thinking about many of the issues and themes which would be eventually conceptualized as American philosophy. Other writers, perhaps most notably William James, grappled with Sanders' line of questioning also, asking what we must do in order to live a significant life. Importantly, both Thoreau and James first asked these questions, and sought these answers, as individuals. Crafting a life of meaning was, for both individuals, anything but merely a theoretical proposition. Both James and Thoreau, like Sanders, harbored a deep sense and need to answer this question on their own terms first.

Sanders writes about the importance of being centered. He underscores the value of cultivating relationships with others as one part of centeredness. Additionally, Sanders (1995) notes that centeredness arises from "inward depths" (ix). Structuring life in a receptive manner occurs through space and time set apart from the world, through times of silence, solitude, and reflection. Centeredness does not necessarily mean stationary, however. In fact, movement may provide the opportune moments for these inward depths to flourish, and provide opportunities to build and foster relationships also. As I run, I experience this quality of centeredness of which Sanders speaks. Running connects me with my surroundings, on occasion with other people (e.g., my running partners), and with myself. My home territory includes moving through spaces like the Lehigh Parkway, past landmarks such as Muhlenberg College, Cedar Beach Park, and Lehigh Valley Hospital. Regardless of the physical space (e.g., my own neighborhood or someplace "new"), running provides this quality of being centered in a way that walking did for Thoreau at Walden.

While vaguely aware of the streams of thought known as transcendentalism and pragmatism as a college student, my first real exposure to American philosophy came during graduate school. Our professor, Doug Anderson (one of the contributors in this work), developed an ethics course (one focused on the broader notion of conduct of life) around the works of Emerson and Thoreau. We spent the semester delving into the writings of both authors and I became increasingly enamored with Thoreau. I discovered—through my writing, personal experiences, and reflection—that a life of simplicity, for example, was not a simple endeavor.

The timing of my doctoral studies coincided with my former role as coach and small-college professor. As I read the transcendentalists, and later the pragmatists, I considered Thoreau's notion of simplicity and wondered, both theoretically and practically, to what extent it was possible for coaches to experience a life of simplicity. I sensed, as Anderson (2006) notes, "the pragmatists—especially James and Dewey—took the Emersonian democratic directive seriously and sought to have American philosophy deal with the everyday experiences from which its questions emerged" (5). This was my connection too, trying to reconcile the challenges of Thoreau's life of simplicity with my then occupation as a college basketball coach (Hochstetler, 1999). I did so unaware I was living out McDermott's (2007) dictum on the importance of making relations, in life and in education. This sense of seeking both meaning and connections continued to develop through my interest in philosophical issues related to endurance sport and, more specifically, running.

It is important to explain my Emersonian angle of vision at the outset. I am a product of southeast Iowa, coming of age during the Farm Crisis of the 1980s, living on a family farm where both work and play counted. I ran in secondary school, inspired by icons such as Frank Shorter, Bill Rodgers, and Alberto Salazar (Salad Bar, my cross-country teammates and I called him), but also encouraged by and ran because of my cousin, Marty, who would eventually win a state cross-country title. Growing up on a farm, surrounded on all sides by Amish neighbors, I ran along gravel roads, past fields of corn and soybeans, one-room schoolhouses, tractors and combines, and away from dive-bombing red-wing blackbirds. Like many of my friends and classmates, I learned the value of hard work through a distinct physicality—by baling hay, loading turkeys, cleaning hog pens, walking beans, and repairing fences. Through these formative experiences I developed an identity based, in part at least, on this farm background and time spent training as an athlete. To some extent these early experiences continue to shape and influence who I am and the lens through which I view the world around me.

There is a certain irony, perhaps, that a small-town, farm boy from Iowa, with a distinctly Midwest background and identity, would become enamored with Thoreau—a writer and thinker from the Northeast who went to Harvard. Remarking on the "anti-intellectualism and . . . distrust of 'impractical,' abstract thinking" found in the Midwest, Mueller (in Pichaske, 2006) contends: "It is unimaginable that, for example, transcendentalism or the art-for-art's sake movement could have arisen in the Midwest" (15). Perhaps Mueller is correct to characterize the Midwest in this way, with suspicion toward intellectualism and value placed in practical and concrete thinking. For example, the state of Missouri identifies as the "Show Me State"—its unofficial nickname. This characterization of Midwesterners as anti-intellectual is surely extremely broad, however, and even a cursory glance at regional demographics demonstrates the spectrum of educational levels (Bureau, U.S. Census, 2017). More to the point, other writers such as Wendell Berry and Scott Sanders describe the importance of experience as a pertinent Midwest theme and value. In this way, my farm background and running experience count as both meaningful and insightful. As such, this corresponds to the notion of experience found in American philosophy such as transcendentalism. Perhaps my resonance with a Northeasterner like Thoreau is not so ironic after all.

## THE AMERICAN PHILOSOPHICAL TRADITION

In his book, *Philosophy Americana*, Doug Anderson (2006) describes American philosophy as "a history—perhaps a natural history—of ideas, persons, and actions that begins, roughly speaking, with the writings of the Mathers and Jonathan Edwards and runs through to the present" (4). It is "American," he continues, "not for jingoistic reasons, but because it is autochthonous—it grows out of the New World environment and experience" (4). In this respect, those ideas and streams of thought arise from a distinctly "American" experience. To live, learn, and grow in Los Angeles or Des Moines or Boston provides a different set of experiences as compared with someone whose life course runs in places like London, rural Sudan, or Quito. While these so-called American experiences may differ from region to region (e.g., Southwest, East) and over time, there remains a certain thread here that is distinct from other places around the world.

In addition to defining American philosophy relative to geography, we might also delineate its form in terms of certain individuals. Writers who typically fall into the American philosophy camp, so to speak, include numerous individuals, many of whom lived in either nineteenth or early twentieth century. For the most part these people lived in the United States, encountering a set of experiences much different from philosophers in other parts of the world. Stuhr (1987), for example, uses the term "classical American philosophy" in reference to influential writers who lived and wrote between approximately 1870 and 1945, including Charles Sanders Peirce, William James, Josiah Royce, George Santayana, John Dewey, and George Herbert Mead. Beyond this list, contributors to this book draw from individuals such as Henry David Thoreau, Ralph Waldo Emerson, and John McDermott, among others. Other notable contributors to American philosophy include females like Jane Addams (a contemporary of Dewey and James) who worked for social reform, and Margaret Fuller (an influential transcendentalist). My own take on American philosophy views the tradition in a big-tent sort of way—with the inclusion of not only academicians and those who self-identify as philosophers but including writers from various backgrounds who speak to issues we refer to as "American" in a clear and insightful manner.

Beyond geography and notable individuals, it is possible to frame the American philosophical tradition in terms of common themes which seem to permeate the writings. Stuhr (1987) posits a number of what he deems to be "defining characteristics and commitments . . . central to the classical American philosophical vision" (5). These include the rejection of modern philosophy; fallibilism; pluralism; radical empiricism; the continuity of science and philosophy; and pragmatism and meliorism (5–9). To elaborate, Anderson (2006) contends that this so-called take on themes consistent with American philosophy includes the following:

> a general outlook regarding the importance of looking forward, the significance of the aesthetic dimensions of experience, the dialectical yet spontaneous interplay of individual and community, the possibility of perceiving meaning and relations and not just discrete atoms of experience, and the fundamental importance of finding and creating the extraordinary in the ordinary. (4)

While this form of "classical American philosophy" has historically focused almost exclusively on white male writers, the tradition has become (finally) more cognizant of the need for increased diversity, with authors who have their own angles of vision—women and individuals of color, for example. Gloria Anzaldúa (2012) is one who drew from her Chicana experiences to give voice to the lives and ideas of those individuals living along the U.S.-Mexico border, and furthermore to those whose lives represent "psychological borderlands, the sexual borderlands, and the spiritual borderlands" (19). Additionally, bell hooks[1] writes from her perspective as a black female from the South. Anderson (2006) writes that hooks' writings "impress us with their autobiographical self-awareness in the absence of self-engrossment or narcissism. For her, philosophy does not mean leaving experience behind. . . . Philosophy must develop *through* one's experiences" (6). Like Henry Bugbee, who contemplates philosophical concepts while in motion—with ideas intimately connected to his experiences (e.g., rowing, swamping, building a dam); and like the endurance athletes and writers whose essays fill these pages; bell hooks and others in the American philosophical tradition lean on their respective experiences, drawing from this inspiration as they think and write.

An additional aspect related to American philosophy regards the overall writing style and approach. Again, while not wholly distinct from other philosophical traditions, some writers have employed a less formal style—one more transitory and open to change. Emerson, for example, used the essay form, here described by Goodman (2015): "The essay—literally a trial or attempt, not a fully finished product or complete system—is the appropriate literary form for a mode of thinking that seeks insights, angles of vision, and progressions of thought, but makes no claim to completeness, nor even at times to correctness" (158). Bugbee (1999) provides another example in *The*

*Inward Morning* which he subtitles: *A Philosophical Exploration in Journal Form*. Bugbee explains his style as such:

> The present day—that is the dwelling of meditative thought. Consequently, this work is in journal form. Not because it is a philosophical notebook or diary; it is neither of these. It is basically a work which required to be done within the day, from the actual human stance which the day might afford, whatever that day might bring. (10)

Bugbee strives to focus his attention on "that day" and the process that enfolds rather than working toward any fixed certainty or sense of closure. Furthermore, Thoreau provides another example of the essay form, as some of his writings appear as journals, with day-by-day accounts and observations interspersed with insightful commentary and philosophical musings. Thoreau (2012) explained the personal nature of his writing this way:

> In most books, the *I*, or first person, is omitted; in this it will be retained; that, in respect to egotism, is the main difference. We commonly do not remember that it is, after all, always the first person that is speaking. I should not talk so much about myself if there were anybody else whom I knew as well. Unfortunately, I am confined to this theme by the narrowness of my experience. (199)

The process of establishing, understanding, and sustaining a body of work and academic field such as American philosophy is a continual challenge. There is an inherent tension between retaining so-called sacred texts— *Walden*, *The American Scholar*, and other influential works written by the nineteenth-century pragmatists and transcendentalists—and the continual creation of other writing that addresses twenty-first century concerns and includes a multiplicity of authors. Emerson spoke to this need for a continual process of renewal, of speaking and writing to one's particular situation. He implored Americans to chronicle their own history and not simply look toward Europe for answers. Stewarding an American philosophical canon of sorts entails an attentiveness toward those writings which continue to define those who identify as Americans, those writings which resonate, challenge, and provide a glimpse of hope.

## THE APPEAL OF AMERICAN PHILOSOPHY

My doctoral studies exposed me to a plethora of philosophical traditions— both Western and Eastern. I found myself drawn to Emerson and Thoreau, in large measure because of their particular stance toward the broader culture, and with my own intent of working in and around other (sport) philosophers of this same ilk. Those individuals thinking and writing as American philosophers do so with hopes of working to make a difference—to make their respective efforts matter or count. As Anderson (2006) writes, "American [philosophers] are hard-core meliorists. We are attentive to the ills around us. We *think* about things; we are committed to goods as ends-in-view.... We are, one might say, *working* utopians" (15). This aspect of working toward something better makes sense to someone brought up in a farm community where making a difference (e.g., planting, harvesting) was important and essential work.

Additionally, philosophy is not limited to abstract notions such as justice, truth, happiness, and so forth, but intersects with and has a bearing on our human endeavors of work and play. Furthermore, as will become much more apparent throughout the course of this book, the themes centrally related to the American philosophical tradition align closely with the challenges and experiences present and faced by runners, cyclists, swimmers, and endurance athletes in general. This is not to say that other philosophical traditions may not intersect with endurance sport—Zen and running comes to mind here, for example. That said, endurance sport and themes from American philosophy are both apparent and important. For example, runners need to ascertain the amount of "truth" present in their marathon training programs (see Sailors and Cash, chapter 7). Cyclists strive to understand how continuing to ride throughout one's life adds to the nature of significance (see Kretchmar, chapter 5). It is entirely possible that other sports—judo or golf or football—relate to American philosophy. However, our task within these pages is distinctly our own—one predicated on and shot through with personal experience. For the writers of these essays, endurance sport provides a lens through which we read, think, and write. Physical activities which include a significant amount of endurance is our existential home and impacts the way we view the world around us.

It seems to me that one of the strengths of this book is the on-the-ground vision that endurance sport participation provides. Through endurance sport—by virtue of hours on the road, trails, and in the water—we may glean insights otherwise left unturned. McDermott (2007) writes: "If we live, think, and act deeply, then we have access to experiences that do not show their hand to a shallow living" (136). Indeed, endurance sport provides ample opportunity for acting deeply. This is consistent with American philosophy in that the seminal writers placed a premium on experience with respect to developing their philosophical positions and values.

Other athletes have their own particular take. We leave those lives (and respective insights) to the basketball players, the divers, and the weight lifters. Accordingly, as Anderson (2006) contends, "we should not abandon our angles of vision and our histories as we apprentice to the philosophical trade. . . . . All of these features of our experiences help constitute the very language of outlooks on the world" (6–7). We need to draw deeply from these experiences to help us understand, and share with others, what it means to live a significant life, how best to navigate the tensions between the individual and community, what it means to commit oneself to a practice (or job, long-term relationship, and so forth). In this way philosophy of sport, as an academic endeavor, benefits from the experiential nature of endurance sport, and sheds light on philosophical issues.

For example, running (and endurance sport in general) might exemplify the dialectical relationship between the individual and the community—when and to what extent to train solo (we all have different levels of needs and places to find our energy) and when and to what extent to engage in community (group runs, partners, races, etc.). Some prefer to run on their own. They may relish this time and experience although perhaps they really need, or at least would benefit from, a modest amount of social contact and connection through group runs. Similarly, one may enjoy the banter of group workouts, but this preference may be at the expense of listening to a personal muse which may appear over time through the solitude of individual runs. Thus, endurance sport provides a vehicle to examine the individual and communal dialectic.

Endurance sport may also exemplify, and perhaps even clarify, the nature of risk and precipitousness. Famously, William James argued for the strenuous life, the importance of taking chances and committing oneself to human projects in the face of tenuous circumstances. Endurance sport athletes live this concept in a visceral way, in their pursuit of improved performance and personal goals as part of their life narrative. As one ultrarunner remarked, "It's about seeing where your ceiling is and realizing it might be higher. Can I go farther? I don't know. It's pushed by a series of I don't knows" (in Hanold, 2016, 187). James (1956), too, held this sentiment and recognized that "Not a victory is gained, not a deed of faithfulness or courage is done, except upon a maybe" (59). One must take those chances, however, in order to complete a marathon, finish an Ironman distance triathlon, or achieve any other endurance sport markers of success. In addition to racing, this might also include those athletes who remain committed to their practice without any need for competition as such.

One challenge for making the connection between endurance sport and philosophy, however, is that this complementary nature must run both ways. This necessitates that those in the endurance sport community recognize or at least entertain the notion that their endeavors might have a philosophical nature; and, that those in the American philosophical tradition understand and appreciate the potential practical wisdom garnered through endurance sport participation. Anderson (2006) puts it this way: "Part of the outlook of American philosophy is the belief that philosophy can be democratic in a rough-and-ready sense. That is, American culture can be brought to philosophy if we philosophers will meet it halfway" (5). Endurance sport demonstrates an affinity for democratic participation—events open to all, regardless of athletic prowess,[2] gender, race, ethnicity, or other characteristics.

In *Walden*, Thoreau (2012) wrote, "To be a philosopher is not merely to have subtle thoughts . . . but so to love wisdom as to live according to its dictates . . . [and] to solve some of the problems of life, not only theoretically, [but] practically" (208–209). In short, rigorous and honest philosophical work requires the complementary pairs of practical and theoretical approaches. This means working toward solving theoretical problems, although not introducing problems just because they are interesting. Rather, the theoretical problems and issues arise within the context of real-world situations and challenges. The authors who write in the following chapters embody this approach as well, writing from their angle of experience as both athletes and academics. Some are formally trained as philosophers and have become interested in sport-related issues; others are schooled in kinesiology and have developed a research line focused on philosophical concepts. In this way the authors represent the cross-disciplinary nature of sport philosophy. This area of academic discourse focuses on how best to understand sport and physical activity vis-à-vis philosophical areas such as metaphysics, axiology, epistemology, aesthetics, and ethics.

## THE NATURE AND APPEAL OF ENDURANCE SPORT

Part of the appeal, at least for me, of American philosophy is its recognition of and appreciation for the seemingly common aspects of human life. Emerson (2009), for example, wrote: "I embrace the common, I explore and sit at the feet of the familiar, the low. Give me insight into to-day, and you may have the antique and future worlds" (57). To run, bike, and swim are in many respects common events. It is not difficult to encounter others (adults, especially) who dedicate themselves to these leisure time pursuits, at least with some level of seriousness. This common nature, the familiarity of running day after day, for example, lends itself to insights available by being on foot, outdoors in the elements. Arguably, the very experience of running outside, as opposed to running on a treadmill for example, is a different one indeed (Hochstetler, 2003). Yet in some ways endurance sport is not common, perhaps in the manner enthusiasts are viewed by the nonparticipant. These individuals might very well regard the endurance runner with curiosity, suspicion or disdain, but conversely, also possibly with respect or admiration. In this way "common" may not be the appropriate term for individuals who complete track workouts at 5 am or run a marathon—after swimming 2.4 miles and cycling 112 miles.³

While perhaps at odds with the normal life of many Americans, the extended time and mundane nature involved with endurance sport activities does lend itself to considerable time for reflection—both of self and one's relationship in community. Goodman (2015) contends that Thoreau's writing in *Economy* "makes us uncomfortable because it pushes us in the direction of a choice about the way we exist in the world. In this respect, Thoreau is as much of an existentialist as his contemporary Soren Kierkegaard" (209). The swimmer who makes turn after turn, lap after lap, over the course of a workout carves out a kind of solitude reminiscent of Thoreau at Walden. To move in this way over an extended period provides opportunity and occasion for musing about one's place in the world. Friedman (2016) captures this notion beautifully with regard to swimming:

> Assuming you have some basic stroke proficiency, your attention is freed from the outside world. You just have to dimly sense the approaching wall before you flip turn and go on your way. Cut off from sound, you are mostly aware of your breathing. You have to traverse boredom before you can get to a state of mental flow. Now your mind is free to revel in nonlinear, associative thought. Nothing has to make sense. You suddenly become aware that time has passed. You are not sure what elapsed in that strange discontinuity, but the solution to a problem that escaped you on land is perfectly obvious emerging from the water—a rapturous experience.

As a lifelong (mostly) runner, experienced (albeit for the most part retired) cyclist, and one with team sport experience in activities ranging from baseball, basketball, football, and soccer, it seems to me the qualities of endurance sport are notably different from other pursuits and, therefore, lend themselves to philosophical reflection in a unique way. It is not my intent here to carve out airtight distinctions between endurance sports and other activities, but rather to draw broad thematic components in a Wittgensteinian family resemblance sort of way. To write a book about endurance sport, therefore, we need at least a cursory understanding of the nature and characteristics of both the activity and those individuals who engage in such activities and identify as endurance athletes.

There is a sense in which the notion of endurance itself may be interpreted as a cultural construct. For example, Adams (2016) wonders, "Out of all the ways to test a body, why test its endurance? . . . There is nothing inherently valuable in the ability to push the body to its physical limits, to keep it moving or to break it down" (32). The Olympic motto of Citius, Altius, Fortius promotes striving for accomplishments which are faster, higher, and stronger—a motto which does not necessarily capture endurance events. Yet our cultural interest in testing endurance feats remains. Endurance sport adherents realize the unique nature of moving for hours at a time. In another place I write, "The experience of 'hitting the wall' during a marathon, for example, is unique to the lived experience specific to these events" (2016, 337).

It may be difficult to describe endurance athletes in general, to ascribe certain characteristics to their nature. That said, former Ironman triathlon winner Scott Tinley (2015) describes endurance athletes as individuals "whose passion for life takes them well beyond the physical and mental confines that imprison others. . . . Endurance athletes are many things but we are not Thoreau's *mass of men living in states of quiet desperation*" (3). The sociological literature aptly describes the broader characteristics of endurance athletes. I use running examples, but the illustrations also extend to other endurance athletes. Beyond the very literal sense in which endurance athletes undergo repetitive movement over time, these activities entail a conscious and very present element of pain. As Anderson and Lally (2004) contend, however, "Not just *any* suffering, pain, or loss will automatically lead to such a clearing for the consideration of ideals. To engage in endurance practices—or any extensive physical training—is to choose a specific sort of physical suffering" (18).

It is possible to delineate various aspects of pain related to endurance sport. For example, some pain suggests injury while other pain does not. Bale (2006) refers to this latter sort of pain as "the deposit, the investment, through which speed is extracted. Pain is a form of bodily or physical capital, a bearer of symbolic value" (66). This form of pain, therefore, is one the endurance athlete puts up with in the context of training and racing. Endurance athletes recognize the nature of pain as a constant presence. They seek not only to tolerate pain, but even to learn from what these sensations can teach—and perhaps even revel in the ability to withstand pain as a badge of honor. Bridel, Markula, and Denison (2016) write, "Pain, thus appears to be part of runners' identity or sense of self: the ability to endure pain, tolerate pain, and/or overcome pain" (7). The ability to endure pain impacts the likelihood of whether or not one ultimately crosses the finish line.

Many endurance athletes (especially ultra-distance athletes) put a premium on finishing races. The primary goal here is not necessarily to win, place, or even garner age-group awards, but rather to keep moving forward to the end. Finishers of the Badwater 135, for example, an event touting itself as the "World's Toughest Foot Race," earn a finisher's T-shirt and belt buckle of distinction to commemorate their finisher's status (badwater.com). As Hockey and Allen-Collinson (2016) write: "Within the distance running subculture, the desire and ability to endure . . . is often juxtaposed with the practice of 'dropping out' of races where the individual ends up in the category of DNF (Did Not Finish)" (229). For the thousands of runners who begin the New York City or Marine Corps Marathons, very few have a realistic chance of attaining victory or even earning an age-group award. Their goal may be "simply" to finish the race or, perhaps, do so in a PR (personal record) fashion.

In order to sustain oneself during training and racing, the endurance athlete must summon up a particular mindset. The athlete may use any number of potential strategies—both associative and dissociative—to cope with the conditions. When the legs feel like lead, and the breathing rate becomes increasingly labored, the endurance athlete needs to counter with helpful strategies; developing the proper mindset is a requisite for success. Hockey and Allen-Collinson (2016) reference the term "digging in" to explain this mentality: "In a distance-running context," they write, "'digging in' means setting one's 'enduring consciousness' (i.e., an enduring frame of mind) to defend the athlete from her/his own frailties in the face of fatigue, discomfort, pain, and a gamut of geographic and climatic stressors" (229). This frame of mind involves a steady resolve to keep going, to stay strong despite the presence of pain and adversity.

## MIDWEST PHILOSOPHICAL THEMES AND WRITERS

Endurance sport has been a constant in my life. My experiences with endurance sport have shaped who I have become and continue to become. Through the course of two cross-country bicycle trips, followed by numerous marathons and countless half-marathons, I have gradually and firmly taken on the identity of a runner (not jogger; see Hopsicker & Hochstetler, 2014) and endurance athlete. In this way, the present topic exemplifies a way to combine my personal and scholarly interests.

Much of my running identity and, more broadly, endurance sport experiences are directly related, in a very rich way, to physical location. My U.S. coast-to-coast bicycle trips covered terrain such as alongside the Grand Canyon rim, through the sweltering Texas summer heat, and ended with a splash in the Atlantic Ocean near Brunswick, Georgia. Similarly, running has brought me in contact with places far and wide—the farmland of rural Iowa, Virginia, and Pennsylvania; the beauty of major cities like Tokyo, London, and Edinburgh.

Similarly, the American philosophical tradition is impacted by and shot through with an experiential nature directly impacted by a sense of place. This specific tradition is American in the sense that it involves individuals and groups of people who live from a specific location—the United States—and during a certain time period. The pragmatists and transcendentalists serve as the forbearers of this tradition, although the genesis of the movements most directly relate to life and experiences in the Northeast. Since then, others have written from and about their own particular region, including places such as Montana (e.g., Henry Bugbee) and the Southwest (e.g., Gloria Anzaldua). Despite their focus on important themes, these individuals do not necessarily represent my own background of intellectual thought in the sense of the Midwest landscape or themes. It is important then for me to delineate a regional sense of American philosophy—a Midwest flavor that resonates with me and represents my intellectual heritage, in the context of endurance sport participation.

William Goyen, a postmodern language poet, once said, "I don't think anyone ever recovers from the place he was born" (in Pichaske, 2006, 6). Though I have spent most of my adult years in Virginia and Pennsylvania, my ties to rural Iowa remain strong and in some respects my birthplace retains a durable hold on my personal identity. As we consider the deep-seated impact of one's geographic location, it also becomes clear that it is common to view others through stereotypical lenses based on regional differences. One (mis)perception is that those who live in rural communities tend to be closed minded and/or insular in nature. While some Midwesterners may in fact transmit these kinds of tendencies, it is also possible that these stereotypes are not entirely accurate. In fact, at their best, Midwesterners who are centered and committed to their lives and land (in a way outlined by Sanders, 1995) may indeed be receptive and open to those who model different lives—those whose cultural, religious, sexual backgrounds are different. Some authors have written about life through their Midwest angle of vision, informed by their geographical location and life experiences. These individuals are in a unique position to comment on life shaped by and through a Midwestern identity.

Thoreau's works impacted Midwest writers, those who focus on nature and agriculture, such as Sanders (2006) in his book *A Private History of Awe:*

> I dated a new era in my life from the reading of Walden. For here was the testament of a man who sought to live a purposeful life, who sensed the fashioning power at work in all that he saw and in his own depths, who never ceased to be astonished by reality, and who strove to record those moments, in the midst of ordinary nature, when he shook with a sense of awe. (203)

In many ways, my own life as a scholar stems from my initial encounter with Thoreau and reading *Walden*. As I pursue various scholarly projects and draw from my own experiences as an endurance athlete, I am continually reminded of many ideas and concepts from his writing.

Perhaps the individual with the most well-known and obvious connections between Midwest strains of thought and classical American philosophy is Wendell Berry. A writer, philosopher, and farmer, Berry was selected to deliver the 2012 Jefferson Lecture in the Humanities sponsored by the National Endowment for the Humanities (NEH). NEH Chairman Jim Leach wrote of Berry: "Tilling the land of his Kentucky forebears, he is a 21st-century Henry David Thoreau" (NEH, 2012). Like Thoreau with his skepticism of "progress" in the nineteenth century, Berry (1996) questions the so-called achievements proclaimed by those in the U.S. Department of Agriculture's (USDA) office. When the USDA refers to the advantageous nature of "economy of size," they mean fewer farmers and larger farms; a recommendation for "specialization"—a focus on many acres planted solely in corn or soybeans, for example, rather than a diversity of agricultural projects and products (36). Both economy of size and specialization have disastrous results, Berry contends, on family farms and the interconnected rural communities.

From my own farm background, I can speak to the forceful pull of governmental initiatives and community pressure toward conformity. During the 1970s, the farm economy in the Midwest went through a boom period, which eventually led to massive expansion of farm operations in places such as rural Iowa. Farmers borrowed money to purchase more land and expensive equipment to till and harvest. When crop prices dropped sharply in the 1980s, bankers became insistent on recalling their loans and many farmers declared bankruptcy. My father, to his everlasting credit, retained his modicum of diversity—raising hogs, cattle, turkeys; growing corn, soybeans, alfalfa— and, by doing so, resisted the drive toward specialization, hyper-growth, and this notion of "progress." While our family struggled financially during this time period, his decision to resist the broader temptation toward expansion and specialization ultimately helped him retain the farm—a farm that had been in his family for over 100 years.

One theme found in Midwest philosophical writings emphasizes a certain rootedness to a physical place. Recognizing the transient nature of contemporary U.S. culture, the tendency to move repeatedly with the optimism of better jobs and relationships elsewhere, Sanders (1995) contends, "The earth needs fewer tourists and more inhabitants, it seems to me—fewer people who float about in bubbles of money and more people committed to knowing and tending their home ground" (16–17). Sanders has in mind the importance of tending one's ground in a literal sense—the fields of corn, wheat, and rye dominating the Midwest landscape. To lose even a small portion of this ground, the topsoil for example, has disastrous economic and environmental consequences. That said, in a broader sense this commitment to location involves tending one's place in a local community, wherever that may be. This attention to one's surroundings runs close to Thoreau's sentiments of Walden and provides a link between my own Midwest farm background and the nature of Thoreau's northeastern rural life.

Writing from his stance as one interested in and committed to sustainable agriculture and environmental issues, Wes Jackson (1996) questioned the wisdom of following the so-called American dream, or pursuing goals measured only in terms of economic success. He chastised the modern university system for offering "only one serious major: upward mobility. Little attention is paid to educating the young to return home, or to go some other place, and dig in" (3). This point is reminiscent of Thoreau, who questioned the notion of "progress"—of new forms of communication (e.g., telegraph) which did not improve the content of the communication itself, or the Gold Rush seekers who chased the allure of quick wealth. Conversely, this notion of commitment, or digging in as Jackson calls it, enables a sense of education of quite another sort—the knowledge which flourishes through long-term relationships. As Sanders (1993) puts it, "Although I have lived in the same region, indeed the same house, for twenty years, I am still discovering what it means to be a citizen" (xv–xvi).

Consistent with Sanders, Berry (2000) pressed a similar point writing, "We should give up the frontier and its boomer 'ethics' of greed, cunning, and violence, and, so near too late, accept settlement as our goal" (136). He went on to argue that colleges and universities would benefit from instruction in "homemaking," for bringing to this sense of settlement the notion that we "now must begin sometimes with remnants, sometimes with ruins" (136). For Berry, we need to settle more, meaning to stay in one place and focus on stability and permanency, foregoing the "boomer" mentality as a result. In her book, *Good Neighbors*, Nancy Rosenblum (2016) contends that the term "settler" connotes "the risk and initial optimism of moving to a new place, of living among unfamiliar people some of whom will, for better or worse, become familiar" (54). The focus becomes placing one's stock in a particular location and group of people, working toward meliorism in an attentive and committed fashion. To live in this committed fashion—in a pragmatic way of working utopians—involves remaining open to new ideas and growth, even though some who settle in rural locations may be perceived otherwise.

Remaining in a constant geographical location confers a sense of depth to one's character and provides opportunities for an intimate look at one's surroundings. The emphasis in Midwestern writing centers on developing an understanding of and appreciation for place. Berry (2000) contends that "We should value familiarity above innovation. Boomer scientists and artists want to discover (so to speak) a place where they have not been. Sticker scientists and artists want to know where they are" (138–139). This sense of familiarity becomes actualized in the lives of endurance athletes. When one runs or bikes or swims over the course of many years, he gains a glimpse of human projects based on this "sticker" mentality. By viewing our endurance sport experiences from a specific geographical position and built day after day over the course of years, we may appreciate all the nuances and perspectives this provides. Knowing where we are as endurance sport athletes, employees and administrators, neighbors and parishioners—by demonstrating our commitment to others we begin to glimpse a sense of self as well. Thus, a "sticker" mentality is beneficial—on the farm, through our endurance sport engagement, and in life in general.

Settling (in the best sense of the word) in a particular location for an extended period of time, and doing so with great attention to one's surroundings, enables an element of intimacy prevalent not only in broader American philosophical streams with writers like Henry Bugbee, but also in Midwest philosophers such as Frederick Kirschenmann (2010). Growing up in the farmlands of North Dakota, Kirschenmann learned an important lesson:

> My father also taught me to be wary of untrammeled objectivity on the farm. Intimacy was also required. My father appreciated objective data that told him, for example, which variety of wheat contained the best yield and quality characteristics. Yet he also had learned that on a real operating farm the highest yields of a particular crop in a given year did not necessarily result in a profitable farm or the farm's long-term survival. (101)

This proximity to the land—paying attention to the soil quality, the moisture level, and so forth—developed over the course of years, enabled his father to make informed decisions in part by art as well as by science. This sense of intimacy applies to endurance sport in similar ways. By virtue of cycling repeatedly, over the course of many years, the cyclist develops a familiarity with her surroundings, sensing when best to push hard during workouts and when, if certain bodily sensations provide feedback, she best tempers her efforts for a given time. This intimacy of the cycling practice, along with knowledge gleaned from the practice community, provides useful information which can be combined with scientific or so-called objective data sources. The cyclist may follow a particular training plan guaranteed to produce the "best results" and yet acknowledge that this in fact may not always happen and, at times, the cyclist might be better off not following this plan, or at least adjusting it slightly to meet her current conditions and needs. The novice may be more inclined to follow her coach without question, while the experienced athlete, like Kirschenmann's father, with years of experiential knowledge is in a better position to adjust training efforts by this sense of art and feel.

The themes of Midwest writers speak to the particular locale of farmland and small-town life, but they are not solely provincial. While Sanders (1995) writes specifically from his Midwest perspective, and about Midwest issues, his "deeper subject is our need to belong somewhere with a full heart, wherever our place may be, whoever our people may be" (ix). This speaks to the importance of becoming immersed in one's surroundings, without the distractions created by self or others. To live in this manner requires attention to one's place, an immersion reminiscent of Bugbee's (1999) narrative accounts of experiences which, for Bugbee give rise to "marrow-bone truth" (42). Sanders' call is not that everyone should move to the Midwest, nor does Thoreau advocate that all should live in the woods. Rather, their message is one promoting a grounded life, one intentionally focused on a given project and community alongside other humans. This does not necessarily lock one into a specific location forever. Yet, it does require a notion of commitment for some extended portion of time. One could be centered in a sense—by traveling constantly—but doing so necessarily gives up the possibility for any long-term investment in a particular place—this is not necessarily good or bad but is a tradeoff nonetheless. For Thoreau, this need to belong somewhere, whether a temporary location such as Walden, or more permanent residency like Concord, allowed him to experience a physical location, to develop an intimacy with the land and the people. He traveled to other locations—to Minnesota, Cape Cod, Katadhin, for example—but kept coming back home.

Endurance sport has the potential to meet "our need to belong somewhere with a full heart" (Sanders, 1995, ix). Running, for example, provides the time and space to spend our energy, to pursue our goals in a way which resonates with who we are. Running and other endurance sports as well provide a sense of belonging, whether that is our place in nature (as in our solitary runs) or our place in the context of other people (as in runs with a training partner or perhaps a running group). In either case, through our endurance pursuits we may feel this sense of belonging. This may be recognizable by the sense of loss when a beloved training partner moves away, or a sense that something is just not right on those "off" days from training.

The American philosophical tradition, perhaps most particularly pragmatism, places a heavy emphasis on meliorism—working toward making things better, the notion that our current model is not perfect and needs perpetual refinement. Yet helping to advance meliorism is a tricky proposition. On the one hand, Sanders (1993) notes, "In our national mythology, the worst fate is to be trapped on a farm, in a village, in the sticks, in some dead-end job or unglamorous marriage or played-out game. Stand still, we are warned, and you die" (105). Yet to make things better requires an investment in and commitment to a specific human project. It requires one to, in a sense, stand still and dig in. This may at times appear, at least to those removed from the situation, as unglamorous or perhaps even as a "dead-end job." The tireless social activism of Dorothy Day comes to mind here, whose labors led to the formation of the Catholic Worker and positive strides for the poor and homeless;

or the social reform efforts of Jane Addams. In this case, the precipitous life advocated by William James may indeed involve staying put, taking the risk to invest oneself to a calling, regardless of the potential notoriety (or lack thereof) involved. A high school coach and teacher, who labors for years at a small, rural school because of a strong commitment to both his career and the students, may be judged by some outsiders as having "settled" in the pejorative sense of the word. Yet for those students and athletes who benefit from his commitment, life is immeasurably better—a clear case of meliorism and working toward an improved life. Yes, in some ways staying put could be viewed as antithetical to meliorism. A good deal of this turns on the attitude of the individual, however. If one perceives the situation as entrapment or a restriction of one's gifts and abilities, then perhaps it is time to pursue other places and projects.

Once the commitment to a particular project is made—to farming, endurance sport, or any other life-giving endeavor—to work toward meliorism requires inordinate amounts of attention. Yet in order to remain attentive, one must temporarily suspend any preconceived notions or ideas. In his journal, Thoreau (1961) wrote:

> It is only when we forget all our learning that we begin to know. I do not get nearer by a hair's breadth to any natural object so long as I presume that I have an introduction to it from some learned man. To conceive of it with a total apprehension I must for the thousandth time approach it as something totally strange. If you would make acquaintance with the ferns you must forget your botany. (210)

To approach our surroundings with an open outlook requires holding together, in tension, a recognition of previous knowledge without allowing this to intrude upon, or cloud, the immediate experience. To use Michael Polanyi's (1977) language, as one becomes more familiar with a specific project (say, riding a bicycle), the subsidiary knowledge fades into the background and one is able to focus on other, more immediate, particulars (Hopsicker, 2010). No longer does one need to focus exclusively on simply staying upright—this skill is ingrained and recedes to the background, allowing the rider to remain open to capture immediate sensations and events, such as reveling in the breath-taking scenery of a fall century ride, or "digging in" to sustain effort in order to finish a particularly difficult stretch of the course or ride.

While a good deal of American ideology mythologizes the wanderer, the conqueror, the explorer, and while there is certainly something to be said for these notions, Sanders and other Midwest writers push toward a committed aspect of a significant life. Sanders (1995) highlights Whitman as an example of this thought process, where: "The net effect of Whitman's rhetoric, if not his biography, was to glamorize the mover at the expense of the settler" (158). Sanders goes on to note prominent American writers for whom place mattered—Thoreau in Massachusetts, Faulkner in Mississippi, Flannery O'Connor in Georgia, and so forth. Midwest writers such as Sanders, Jackson, and Berry follow this move as well, writing from their own angle of vision from the rural and central portions of the United States.

In part, the aim of this book is to help unpack this potential for endurance sport. We need to understand more fully how giving oneself to endurance sport happens experientially, and what this form of commitment means for our lives and for the lives of others with whom we come into contact. Yes, we may experience setbacks and unfulfilled goals as a result of our endurance sport commitments, but this is the case for any commitment. In the following chapters, the authors provide many insights into their lives as endurance athletes, and scholars who care deeply and have thought carefully about endurance sport and its intersection with philosophic ideas. Beyond an intellectual opportunity, however, I hope this book reaffirms your own movement-related experiences—endurance sport, perhaps—but more broadly any exposure to and commitments toward a specific form of sport and physical activity. I invite you to ponder how these experiences enhance your own understanding of and appreciation for lives of significance and meaning.

## NOTES

1. Born Gloria Jean Watkins, hooks uses this pen name and its lowercase form to honor her maternal great-grandmother.
2. Some ultras require participants to qualify based, in part, for health and safety concerns. The Boston Marathon also requires qualification times although some runners take part to help sponsor nonprofit causes.
3. Beyond these examples, endurance sport enthusiasts have developed even longer tests of endurance—the Quintuple Anvil Triathlon, for instance, where competitors attempt to complete five Ironman-length races in five consecutive days.

## REFERENCES

Adams, M.L. (2016). "Astounding exploits" and "laborious undertakings": Nineteenth-century pedestrianism and the cultural meanings of endurance. In Bridel, W., Markula, P., & Denison, J. (Eds.), *Endurance running: A socio-cultural examination*, 19–34. Abingdon, UK: Routledge.
Alexander, H.B. (1919). *Letters to teachers*. Chicago, IL: Open Court Publishing.

Anderson, D. (2006). *Philosophy Americana: Making philosophy at home in American culture*. New York, NY: Fordham University Press.

Anderson, D., & Lally, R. (2004). Endurance sport. *Streams of William James*, 6(2), 17–21.

Anzaldúa, G. (2012). *Borderlands/La Frontera*. San Francisco, CA: Aunt Lute Books.

Bale. (2006). The place of pain in running. In Loland, S., Skirstad, B., & Waddington, I. (Eds.), *Pain and injury in sport: Social and ethical analysis*, 65–75. New York, NY: Routledge.

Berry, W. (1996). *The unsettling of America: Culture & agriculture*. San Francisco, CA: Sierra Club Books.

Berry, W. (2000). *Life is a miracle*. Washington, DC: Counterpoint.

Bridel, W., Markula, P., & Denison, J. (2016). Critical considerations of runners and running. In Bridel, W., Markula, P., & Denison, J. (Eds.), *Endurance running: A socio-cultural examination*, 1–15. London, UK: Routledge.

Bugbee, H. (1999). *The inward morning*. Athens, GA: University of Georgia Press.

Bureau, U.S. Census. American FactFinder—Results. factfinder.census.gov. Retrieved 2017-01-19.

Emerson, R. (2009). *The essential writing of Ralph Waldo Emerson*. New York, NY: Random House.

Friedman, Richard A. Pool of Thought. New York Times Online, last modified July 16, 2016. http://www.nytimes.com/2016/07/17/opinion/sunday/pool-neuroscience.html?ref=opinion&_r=0

Goodman, R. (2015). *American philosophy before pragmatism*. Oxford, UK: Oxford University Press.

Hanold, M. (2016). Ultrarunning. In Bridel, W., Markula, P., & Denison, J. (Eds.), *Endurance running: A socio-cultural examination*, 181–194. Abingdon, UK.

Hochstetler, D. (2007). Can we experience significance on a treadmill? In Austin, M.W. (Ed.), *Running & philosophy: A marathon for the mind*, 139–149. Malden, MA: Blackwell Publishing.

Hochstetler, D., & Hopsicker, P. (2016). Normative concerns for endurance athletes. *Journal of the Philosophy of Sport*, 43(3), 335–349. doi:10.1080/00948705.2016.1163226.

Hockey, John, and Jacquelyn Allen-Collinson. (2015). "Digging in: The sociological phenomenology of "doing endurance" in distance-running." In *Endurance Running*, 227–242. Routledge.

Hooks, B. (1990). *Yearning: Race, gender, and cultural politics*. Boston, MA: South End Press.

Hopsicker, P.M. (2010). Learning to ride a bike. In Ilundáin-Agurruza, Jesús, & Michael W. Austin (Eds.), *Cycling-Philosophy for Everyone: A Philosophical Tour de Force*, 16–26. Wiley-Blackwell.

Hopsicker, P.M., & Hochstetler, D. (2014). Finding the 'Me' in endurance sports: An apology for runners & joggers and cyclists & riders. *Kinesiology Review*, 3, 161–171.

Jackson, W. (1996). *Becoming native to this place*. Washington, DC: Counterpoint.

James, W. (1956). *The will to believe: And other essays in popular philosophy.* Mineola, NY: Dover Publications.

Kirschenmann, F. (2010). *Cultivating an ecological conscience: Essays from a farmer philosopher.* Lexington, KY: The University of Press of Kentucky.

McDermott, J. (2007). *The drama of possibility: Experience as philosophy of culture.* Edited by Douglas R. Anderson. New York, NY: Fordham University Press.

National Endowment for the Humanities. http://www.neh.gov/news/press-release/20 12-02-06.

Pichaske, P. (2006). *Rooted: Seven Midwest writers of place.* Iowa City, IA: University of Iowa Press.

Polanyi, M., & Prosch, H. (1977). *Meaning.* University of Chicago Press.

Rosenblum, N. (2016). *Good neighbors: The democracy of everyday life in America.* Princeton, NJ: Princeton University Press.

Sanders, S. (1993). *Staying put: Making a home in a restless world.* Boston, MA: Beacon Press.

Sanders, S. (1995). *Writing from the center.* Bloomington, IN: Indiana University Press.

Sanders, S. (2006). *A private history of awe.* New York, NY: North Point Press.

Stuhr, J. (1987) (Ed.). *Classical American philosophy.* New York, NY: Oxford University Press.

Thoreau, H. (1961). *The heart of Thoreau's journals.* Edited by Odell Shepard. Dover Publications.

Thoreau, H. (2012). *The portable Thoreau.* Penguin.

Tinley, S. (2015). *Finding triathlon: How endurance sports explain the world.* Hobart, NY: Hatherleigh Press.

Vitek, B., & Jackson, W. (Eds.). (2008). *The virtues of ignorance: Complexity, sustainability, and the limits of knowledge.* Lexington, KY: The University Press of Kentucky.

*Chapter 1*

# Running and Musing
## *Living Philosophically*
### Douglas Anderson

If one queries Google about the relationship between endurance running and thinking, the first several pages of responses are filled with the ways one can adjust one's thinking to improve one's performance. There are also a number of entries from *Huffington Post* and elsewhere citing Ashley Samson's July 2015 study of "elite runners" published in the *International Journal of Sport and Exercise Psychology* that maintains that runners spend about 40 percent of their running time thinking about distance and pacing and that 32 percent of their thoughts attend to their suffering and pain. I have run and cycled with such folks; and they are often elite athletes. They carry watches and keep logs of miles and meals. I have no quarrel with these folks, but I am not one of them. The cash value of my running is somewhat different than theirs. As Kathryn Schulz (2015) points out in "What We Think about When We Run," from a more general consideration of running, Samson's study misses the point. It depends on who the "we" is. Many of us who run long distances think of many things.

    The Google search reveals the obvious. We who study philosophies and sciences of sport most often try to make sense of what we do in sport and, on the practical side, we try to figure out how we can improve our performances. Much university research is driven by the "improvement" model. And running magazines, much like golf magazines, routinely explore the newest ways to gain some minimal advantage. A quick look at the last year of *Runner's World*, for example, reveals articles on improving motivation, using squats to improve sprinting, and increasing speed through short rest workouts. We scholars also ask occasionally what running can do for us. Much of this sort of inquiry assesses the health and practical life benefits of running. Again, I do not mean to be dismissive of these various studies. But in the essay at hand, I want to turn the tables just a bit and ask not what philosophy and social science can do for running nor what running can do for my physical well-being, but what endurance running can do for philosophy. More specifically, how might distance running enable reflective thought and, on a larger scale, how might it help us engender a philosophical life? I have here in mind what the Greeks, and more recently Pierre Hadot (2002), understood philosophy to be: "Above all, philosophy was viewed as an exercise of wisdom, and therefore as the practice of a way of life" (49). In general, this is an outlook that was shared by the three originary pragmatists: Charles Peirce, William James, and John Dewey. As Dewey sometimes put it, philosophy should deal not just with the problems of philosophers but also with the problems of persons. Most commentators have understood this about James and Dewey; fewer realize that, in the end, Peirce's own theoretical work was driven both by experiential underpinnings and an interest in the pragmatic meanings of ideas and human habits.

Let's begin this brief journey on running and musing, then, with a short section from Peirce's (1998) last published essay, entitled "A Neglected Argument for the Reality of God." The essay does take up the question of "God's reality" in the peculiar way that Peirce understood that phrase. But the essay was also a final opportunity for Peirce, whose work was generally ignored by the emerging "profession" of philosophy, to provide an overview of his fifty years of philosophical engagement. He understood human reflection as a natural phenomenon that often involved inquiry—looking for ways to find new answers to our existential human doubts. At the beginning of the reflective process of inquiry he placed an attitude of mental playfulness that he called "musement." Peirce famously moved past the traditional logical dichotomy of deduction (necessary reasoning) and induction (probabilistic reasoning), adding a third logical mode which he named variously abduction, hypothesis, and retroduction (plausibilistic reasoning). Discussion of abduction has become extremely popular in the last ten to twenty years in all fields. Folks have finally again become interested, as was Aristotle, in how we come to the premises by which we live. This initial moment of inquiry is where we begin to generate our possible and plausible answers to our questions. And this mode of logicality, Peirce argued, benefited from an experiential attitude of musement. That is, the practice of musing is the chief way we humans creatively find hypothetical answers to the questions that face us—questions of all kinds, from theoretical physics to the best way across town. Peirce, contrary to what some have argued, was not offering a reductive psychological story of the human mind; on the contrary, he aimed to provide an experiential, or phenomenological, glimpse into the general outlook and method of humans looking to creatively answer questions. My addendum to Peirce's account of musement is simple—for some human animals, endurance running is one of the best catalysts for a musing attitude. But I must back up a bit.

Peirce never intended his accounts of abduction and musement to be original; if ideas are too original, he believed, they are likely to be false. He traced many of his ideas on inquiry directly to Aristotle and to Socrates. He believed that, if one looked closely, examples of abduction and musement were to be found throughout the history of western thought, even if they were unarticulated. Meditative and contemplative practices were important for the Greek, Roman, Judaic, and Christian philosophical traditions. "Meditation," and its Greek root *meléte* (named from one of the three Greek Muses), referred to a variety of practices from verbal and silent recitation to repetition of a physical action to internal reverie. What these practices had in common was the effect of altering the mind's attitude and orientation. For Plato, at least on a few occasions (e.g., Sophist 263, 4e), meditation—or "thinking"—meant attention to internal dialogue or reflection, and it is this mode of meditation that I have in mind when I consider endurance running. And it was the basis, I think, for Peirce's development of musement. The habits of reflection and attentiveness to our experiences are, for me, the very foundation of living philosophically. Here again I align myself with Hadot (2002) and his understanding of Greek thought:

> "the philosopher," he noted, "will never attain wisdom, but he [she] can make progress in its direction. According to the *Symposium*, then, philosophy is not wisdom, but a way of life and discourse determined by the *idea* of wisdom." (46)

Endurance running is, for me, a practice that engenders attention to musement and reflection, and, as an ongoing practice in life, may be one avenue for learning how to live philosophically.

## RUNNING AND MUSING

Charles Peirce was a working scientist and a first-rate logician and mathematician. As we look back through the lens of twentieth-century professional philosophy with its narrow focus on linguistic analysis, it seems unusual that he should build his last public essay around his notion of musement. Through this lens, this is perhaps something one would expect from William James or Henri Bergson but not from Peirce. Indeed, many commentators have tried to separate this experiential side of Peirce from his more technical logical work; but this separating activity tells us more about the commentators than it does about Peirce. Peirce's experiential side and his focus on musement and the creative development of hypotheses was a feature of his work throughout his career. It appeared throughout his youthful jottings and in his earliest published pieces in the 1860s. To initiate my exploration of running and musing,

I will mine Peirce's (1998) long passage on musement from this final essay for what I take to be several key features.

I begin with part of the opening of the passage:

> There is a certain agreeable occupation of mind which, from its having no distinctive name, I infer is not as commonly practiced as it deserves to be; for indulged in moderately,—say through some five to six percent of one's waking time, perhaps during a stroll,—is refreshing enough more than to repay the expenditure. (Peirce, 436)

My own one- to two-hour daily run fits well into Peirce's 5–6 percent range. And it is important to note that the practice of musement is not only useful for creative and abductive thinking but is also "refreshing." Indeed, I would amend Peirce's point to say that it can be refreshing not only in its aftermath but also in its presence.

Following the spirit of his youthful reading of Friedrich Schiller's *Aesthetic Letters*, Peirce (1998) says of musement, "In Fact, it is Pure Play. Now, Play, we all know, is a lively exercise of one's powers" (436). Musement is thus a kind of activity—one's mind is alive, not deadened. We are using our mental abilities. But our exercise of mental powers should not be aligned with or be mistaken for domination and control. Play involves a relinquishing of over-control—it is free, not too serious, and easygoing. Schiller (1965) aptly describes the experiential situation; play is "the extinction of time within time" (74). The pure play of ideas requires a playful attitude in which we allow ideas to work through us; to muse is to actively become receptive to the insistence of our ideas. When I begin a long run, I usually think about the initial stiffness of my body or the difficulty of the first climb, but, as my body settles into the run, my mind freely moves away from bodily concerns and begins its own journey. It is here that I depart from elite runners and those whose focus is some mode of competition with others or with one's own previous times. It is here that we reap different benefits from our running.

I do not begin by forcing myself to think of anything in particular; indeed, if I do occasionally do so, I do not muse, but exercise my mental powers in a much more mechanical and directed way. Instead, I allow ideas that perhaps have been in waiting during my daily routines to make their presence known. As Henry Bugbee (1999) put it: "Nothing can be truly given to us except on the condition of active receptiveness on our part" (133). I am, in Emersonian fashion, at the whim of the ideas themselves and "thinking" may take any number of forms, from imagining to projecting to poetizing to calculating. For Peirce (1998), musement "may take either the form of aesthetic contemplation, or that of distant castle-building (whether in Spain or within one's own moral training), or that of considering some wonder in one of the Universes [of experience] or some connection between two of the three, with speculation concerning its cause" (436).[1] In short, Peirce did not wish to constrain how our minds might work while musing. One of the things I have found a long run can do is enable the "letting go" of control of my mental activity, thus allowing the play of musement to take hold. This is why meditation, regardless of its mode or its catalyst, is an art and not a science; we are not actively in control of the experimentation that occurs. There is no mechanical recipe for meditating; we must learn it in practice. At the same time, as a *techne*, "letting go" (meditating) is not random or chaotic; we learn it *as* a practice. The art is in learning how to let go and to let ideas play freely.

This is not to say, however, that it is not possible to "seed" musement in the way one might seed a dream. Occasionally, I will take a run when I am working on an outline or when I get stuck on the verse of a song. On some of those occasions the outline ideas or verse possibilities will appear as I run. But at other times, even when I have laid the groundwork, my mind will not attend to these but will play with ideas about the origin of the universe or the meaning of particular memories. The point is that the muser is at play and does not actively choreograph the dance of ideas. Peirce (1998) points to the difference in considering religious beliefs:

> One who sits down with the purpose of becoming convinced of the truth of religion is plainly not inquiring in scientific singleness of heart, and must always suspect himself [or herself] of reasoning unfairly. . . . But let religious meditation be allowed to grow up spontaneously out of Pure Play without any breach of continuity; and the Muser will retain the perfect candor proper to Musement. (436)

This is why, for Peirce, specific texts and creeds are more likely to inhibit religiosity than to inspire it; and this is why religious belief is for him both vague and general and is not tied to specific historical doctrines. This is also the reason I do not tend to count Descartes' *Meditations* as genuine meditations or musings. Descartes eventually returned to the very beliefs he claimed to doubt and to leave behind—it seems more like controlled calculation than meditative musing.

Because musing requires a letting go of simple logical and mental control, it can be catalyzed but it cannot be dictated. Peirce (1998) therefore offers generic advice for enabling the play of musement, and I want to explore several features of this advice in conjunction with my own focus on endurance running. He first mentions "timing": "The dawn and the gloaming most invite one to Musement; but I have found no watch of the nychthemeron that has not its own advantage for the pursuit" (436). He suggests that the transition periods of the day are most inviting—dawn and twilight. I think many runners will agree. Early morning when the world is silent creates a mental and physical space that enables receptivity; likewise, twilight is fueled by the day's activities but is no longer directly entangled with them. There is a freshness in the early day before the business of life and a refreshingness in a late afternoon run. But he is also right to suggest that any time of day might work; not everyone lives by the same clock. Many of us switch our body-clocks from time to time. Timing depends in large part on the runner's and muser's particular situation at a particular time. For example, I find sunset runs often inspire musement; their vibrant beauty takes me away from daily affairs and sets my mind adrift in aesthetic contemplation. And sometimes I find a late night run will lead to playful reflection. I find, for example, that hills are much easier to handle in the dark when I cannot see the incline; my mind is freed from attention to the run itself. The flexibility of timing occurs, however, not just because of the person involved but also because the environments in which we find ourselves are always shifting.

Peirce's (1998) second moment of advice, metaphorically presented, has to do with place and environment:

> Enter your skiff of Musement, push off into the lake of thought, and leave the breath of heaven to swell your sail. With your eyes open, awake to what is about and within you, and open conversation with yourself; for such is all meditation. (437)

The idea of being adrift in our skiff is at work here. There is much to unpack. Two landscapes emerge in our musing—the inner terrain of our moods, memories, and thoughts, and the outer terrain of the environments in which we find ourselves. Both require attention, and it is when they work in complementary fashion that musing and creativity most often ensue.

Consider first how we talk about ourselves and our minds. We ask, "where is your head at?" We say someone is "out to lunch" or "spaced out." We have a wealth of language for the inner terrain built on metaphors from and analogies to outer terrains. We say folks are "crooked" or "mixed up"; we say they are "sweet" or "beautiful" in soul. We all experience ourselves through such analogies and metaphors. The world of musement has its own conditions—we must be "open" and "receptive." A muser must also be "patient"—from a Latin root for suffering, bearing, or undergoing. Our inner terrain is crucial to the development of musing. "I would suggest," Peirce (1998) says, "that the Muser be not too impatient" (438). The Muser, he says, must also not be too "serious"—from a Latin root for heaviness. In short, the frame of mind of the Muser—patient and light—is crucial to the possibility of musing—and this, for me, is why distance running is such a natural catalyst; it has the capacity to reframe my mind.

The outer terrain becomes significant in part because the inner terrain begins to attend to it. I offer a small sample from my own running experiences. One late-afternoon autumn run took me past sets of corn-stubbled fields. My thoughts drifted from the red-brown of the fields in the fading sunlight to the feeling of the harvest, and then to corn-mash, to living alone in the forest beyond the fields. As these thoughts were at play, the haunting, almost melancholic mood of autumn was also present. The inner and outer terrains began working in concert. As a result, lyrics began to appear together with music, and to self-generate in the rhythm of my running, and a song—later named "Mason Jar Whiskey"—was born in its incipiency. On my return home, with the spell of musement past, I was able to bring back enough of the musing to begin the work of crafting the song. But the "hypothesis"—the abductive, creative moment—occurred in the musing on the run. We sometimes like to say our ideas "came out of nowhere." I am more inclined to think, with Peirce, that they are enabled, catalyzed, and partly engendered by the confluence of time, place, and attitude in a musing that was, in the present case, the result of a long distance run—perhaps about ten miles on that occasion.

Another song was born from a run that took me past a local riverbed of dried sand as a result of several weeks of drought. Already in a state of musement, my eyes were drawn to the riverbed and I imagined being drunk and destitute, lying face down in the sand. Place-time—feelings took on a musing ride through the imaginative experience of a wayward alcoholic. The song, "Bone Dry River," grew from the musement experience. I offer the examples of the songs because they are reasonably easy to describe in outline form, but some of my running musings have undertaken to answer some of the most complex interpretive and philosophical problems I have encountered. In the depths of a recent run, I was musing on the nature of Peirce's famous three categories: firstness, secondness, and thirdness. These categories, in their formal structure and their vague experiential associations, present a wonderful puzzle for Peirce scholars. It occurred to me as I was running that Peirce had provided a community of inquirers for logic and science and a community of love for moral considerations, but he never described a community for aesthetics or beauty. The rest of the run involved a sophisticated musing on what such a community might be like and from the musings a paper developed. I do not claim universality, or even generality, for these kinds of experience of running and musing, but I am convinced that at least some others will have experienced the catalyzing effect of distance running for creative musing. And that, for me, is enough to show that running may on occasion be beneficial to the practice of philosophizing.

## RUNNING AND LIVING PHILOSOPHICALLY

While I am convinced experientially of the complementariness of running and musing on specific occasions, I was a long time coming to the realization that there was another dimension to this complementariness. For many years—perhaps twenty-one at this point—I have made an effort to run at least four miles every day. I have done so not to lose weight, not to gain fitness, but just to run. One of the long-term effects is that through the running I have created a habit of musing. I am well aware of the stress-relief and other benefits of a running practice, and I am also aware of the many dangers. But I run to run and have found that in the process I have become more reflective about every aspect of my life. Here I am in full agreement with Bugbee (1999) whose movement is walking not running:

> During my years of graduate study before the war I studied philosophy in the classroom and at the desk, but my philosophy took shape mainly on foot. It was truly peripatetic, engendered not merely while walking, but *through* walking that was essentially a *meditation of place*. And the balance in which I weighed the ideas I was studying was always that established in the experience of walking in the place. (139)

Our philosophies are not sets of propositions laid out in neat rows; they are ongoing musings of meanings that reveal life's losses and importances.

In musing, I am repeatedly brought into self-encounter and, at some moments, self-aversion. The long hard run, as my former running partner Rich Lally used to say, "strips away" the layers of the self and lays us bare to ourselves. We noted earlier that Peirce saw musement as a conversation with oneself. Like Socrates, this is what he took thinking to be at its root—a dialogue of self with self. However, Peirce (1998) was insistent that this sort of conversation is never limited to conventional language. "It is," he says, "not a conversation in words alone, but is illustrated, like a lecture, with diagrams and experiments" (437). When I attend carefully to the reflections in my musings, I do not think this point can be emphasized enough. We live amidst a wide variety of signs, interior and exterior. The receptivity of musings includes not only conventional words and ideas, but also images, memories, sounds, feelings, hues, relations, Jamesian flights and perchings, and the melding of all of these into each other. It is an ongoing complex and comprehensive reflection on the meanings of one's life. It is a thick mode of experience and will never be fully grasped through analysis, which is why, I think, both James and Peirce took to metaphorical, experiential expression. Such expression brings us closer to the experiences than does any analysis of language. We live in our habits, and running and musing allows us to explore, remodel, and recreate these habits when they reveal questions to us—it is the condition of our self-transcendence.

In western traditions, meditative practices were intended to be transformative—they were an avenue to what Emerson sometimes called self-transcendence. I cannot think of a better way to characterize my running/musing habit; it has enabled me to confront myself, to see myself for good and ill, and it has many times opened new roads for life to travel. But I need to be careful here. I am not suggesting a recipe for "the good life" and neither was Peirce. I think "good lives" appear in many guises. What the habit has done for me is to allow me to experiment with my life in the effort to make it a better life. Running/musing has been for me an ameliorative practice. Whatever one's road is to a reflective, ameliorative practice, I believe it is important in life to have such a road. Its absence is, I believe, at the heart of what Thoreau called "lives of quiet desperation."

The habit of running/musing has, for me, been a road out of routinized and mechanized life. The range of reflection is remarkable—from the insanely beautiful as when running in late August I begin to muse on the beauties of the various butterflies that litter the pathway of my run to the hauntingness of the bone dry river bed, and from the personally psychological to the cosmically communal. When Hadot characterizes living philosophically as pursuing wisdom even as we remain aware of and awake to our finitude and fallibility, I think we cannot do better. The profession of philosophy has given itself over to analytic puzzles and a hardened resistance to meditative and contemplative experiences. These are ridiculed as "new age" or more formally as "psychologizing." But the forgetfulness of the experiences of meditating and musing has been a disaster for the relevance of philosophy to the issues of everyday human existence. As enjoyable as solving a puzzle is, it does little to bring wisdom to life. And so, in my habit of running and musing, I side with the amateurs, those who find themselves seeking wisdom in body and spirit—those who seek not to the find "*the* meaning of life" but to find meanings in their particular and shared lives. Running may be beneficial to us in a wide variety of ways; in bringing me to a habit of musement, it has enabled me to begin to live philosophically.

## NOTE

1. Peirce is well known for his three phenomenological and ontological categories: firstness, secondness, and thirdness. When he applied these to experience generally, he identified three "universes" of experience: the universe of ideas, the universe of brute actuality, and the universe of mediation or signs.

## REFERENCES

Bugbee, Henry. (1999) *The Inward Morning*. Athens: University of Georgia Press.

Hadot, Pierre. (2002) *What Is Greek Philosophy?* Trans. Michael Chase. Cambridge: Harvard University Press.

Peirce, Charles. (1998) *The Essential Peirce: Volume 2*. Ed. Nathan Houser. Bloomington: Indiana University Press.

Samson, A., Simpson, D., Kamphoff, C., & Langlier, A. (2015) Think aloud: An examination of distance runners' thought processes. *International Journal of Sport and Exercise Psychology*, 1–14. doi: 10.1080/1612197X.2015.1069877.

Schiller, Friederich. (1965) *On the Aesthetic Education of Man*. Trans. R. Snell. New York: Ungar.

Schulz, Kathryn. (2015) What we think about when we run. *New Yorker*, http://www.newyorker.com/news/sporting-scene/what-we-think-about-when-we-run.

*Chapter 2*

# When Continentalism Meets Pragmatism

## *Enduring Life in the Strenuous Mood*

Ron Welters

### PROPER GEAR

Philosophy is often epitomized as the noble but shy art of asking the right questions.[1] Here I will try to formulate at least some idea of a tangible answer to the matter of how we are to live in times of alleged moral disorientation. Rooted in continental philosophy, but simultaneously beguiled by the pragmatic adage that truth only can be found in the practical consequences of philosophical thinking, I will argue in favor of a fully lived strenuous endurance sport life by referring to both traditions, which I perceive as complementary rather than exclusionary. Endurance sport, performed in depth and width, and conceived as a committed and holistic lifestyle, rather than a gratuitous playful pastime, is a preferential tool for carving the good lives we are to lead into a sustainable future.

As for my continentally based view on the benefits of human endurance in general, I am indebted to the contemporary German philosopher Peter Sloterdijk (1947). Although well established in Immanuel Kant's transcendental idealism,[2] and strongly influenced by the ominous writings of Friedrich Nietzsche (1844–1900) and Martin Heidegger (1889–1976), Sloterdijk's autonomous, exuberant, literary eclectic, and at times elusive work is hard to grasp in terms of a specific philosophical school or style. Still, if one were to determine an overarching theme in Sloterdijk's thoughts, this at best could be described as an ongoing attempt to address societal issues in an evocative style with at times explicit hints at possible directions for improving our lives.

In *You Must Change Your Life—On Anthropotechnics* (2013) Sloterdijk argues that self-improvement through repetitive practice (*askesis*) is the key theme of human existence since time immemorial.[3] Our ascetic planet is inhabited by individuals who are constantly and relentlessly training themselves for the better. This may be self-focused, in the sense that a dedicated practicing may lead to an individual radical lifestyle turn, or *metanoia*. But it may also have a broader scope: we train ourselves to become better humans, contributing to a better society. Ideally this literally results in a "renaissance": a collective rebirth of a forgotten or neglected lifestyle.

Sloterdijk's broadly oriented conception of "anthropotechnics"—roughly all kinds of refined human practices developed over time that safeguard and optimize life, from sheep-herding to biotechnology—resembles the pragmatic notion of "meliorism": the belief that the world tends to get better as a result of human efforts. Jonathon Kahn (2009) contends that this usually refers to the idea of "society's innate, inexorable tendency toward improvement" (37). This is a naturalistic fallacy, which resembles Adam Smith's invisible hand. In addition, Kahn seems to have second thoughts. He therefore proposes William James' specific pragmatic variant of meliorism in which the idea of human-made hope as a more obvious enhancer for the desirable societal change comes to the fore.

In addition, Sloterdijk apparently cherishes a hope for betterment through active anthropotechnical intervention. In *You Must Change Your Life* explicit references to James are sparse, however. Sloterdijk's idea of well-understood and well-performed training programs has a stronger connection with pragmatic ponderings, however. Following the pragmatist stance on endurance sport developed by Douglas Hochstetler and Peter M. Hopsicker (2012), I will argue that we, in order to grasp the full meaning of endurance sport, and to reach for the Aristotelian ideal of *eudaimonia*, or human flourishing, have to become true runners and real cyclists rather than dabbling joggers and occasional weekend warriors, indeed. Although the authors contend that there can or perhaps even should be seasons of life when athletes engage in endurance sport in a monomaniac manner, they warn of "the potential dark side of this pursuit of excellence" (2016, 335), becoming a technical obsession and relinquishing other interests. To carve out "an Aristotelian Golden Mean of sorts between minions and puny fellows" (336), they argue for a proper balance between an extreme dedication to endurance sport, on the one hand, and taking care of relationships and social responsibilities, on the other.

I will develop a more individualistic, even somewhat anti-social take on endurance sport as a preferential tool for strenuously materializing the ideal of human flourishing. Decidedly developing one's very own personal "vertical challenge" codes paradoxically may be the incentive for the more durable lifestyle we need on the collective level. We need to push ourselves uncompromisingly to our very limits for a better world. Sloterdijk's specific continentalism and a lived through variant of pragmatism will go hand in hand when it comes to understanding a sporty life fully lived in endurance. A practical and practicable philosophy that provides some idea of an answer to how we are to live, that is the heart of the strenuous matter.

Before slowly starting to pedal for durable meaning, two more considerations are in order. First, one should note that Sloterdijk is also a practitioner of the strenuous kind himself. Being a runner in his younger days he later changed to cycling, which for him represents the modern variant of ancient heroism. Especially the vertically challenged climber who, ahead of the pack, leaves all mortals far behind, deserves our respect as a contemporary substitute of the ancient god-athlete. Gorris and Kurbjuweit (2008) contend that "anyone can fight on flat stretches, but those who remain capable of fighting a duel on the worst of mountains already deserve to be called Hector or Achilles."

Sympathizing with Heidegger's famous remark on the indeterminateness of *Das Man* ("the they" or "the one:" "Everyone is the other, and no one is himself" (2008, 165)) in our ordinary use of language, finally also a short note on my own practical philosophical gear that helps me to channel my fluttering thoughts. I own and frequently use seven bicycles—ranging from a rickety city-bike to a high-end meticulously maintained time-trial machine—and currently five pairs of running shoes. (I do not possess a driver's license, however.) Recently, I also took up swimming, so I can finally step over from long distance duathlon to the real thing: the ironman distance triathlon, preferably a rather mountainous one. I spend my time swimming in a lake (and shortly hopefully in the sea), running in the woods and cycling uphill, at my own pace and occasionally striving for my personal best or even a podium place in my age-group race. But mostly training. Preferably in a small group or often simply on my many voiced own. Combining preaching with practicing, that is what makes my philosophical life worthwhile.

## BLURRING LIMITS

Still in the neutral zone before the real start, we should have a closer look at the state of the contemporary academic sport philosophy discipline. In *The Grasshopper: Games, Life and Utopia,* the Canadian philosopher Bernard Suits (1925–2007) put forward an often-cited portable definition for game-playing as "a voluntary attempt to overcome unnecessary obstacles" (2005, 54). As a follow-up for the witty grasshopper, who refused to work for winter supplies, since he considered uncommitted play to be his very essence, over time Suits developed a more refined heuristic framework. First, he discerns the innate human urge to play. Games, then, are formally condensed forms of play. Moreover, sports, finally, are competitive, rule-bound games. Suits coined the term "tricky triad" to describe these three partly overlapping notions: "Games and sports are enterprises or institutions, I suggest, in which the exhibition of skill is the paramount consideration, and I'm going to argue that in play the exhibition of skill is not the paramount consideration" (1988, 1).

Following Suits' claims, contemporary narrow internalists, or formalists, still work up the axiom that games are solely defined by their rules. Broad internalists, or interpretivists, on the other hand, contend that there is an intrinsic ethos in sport that reaches beyond sheer rules: the "spirit" of sports, expressed in the call for fair play or the willingness to play a game beautifully, and not just to win it. Over the years externalism has gained more influence, however. According to this "heterotelic" stance sports are not just playful, or "lusory," self-referential ends in themselves, but to some extent inevitably are always also means to other ends. Say prestige, power, and prize-money on the cynical side of the spectrum and sport as a health-enhancer and social glue on the other.

So, in the academic philosophy of sport there are two different styles of approaching the subject matter: the precise and the amenable basic attitude, the so-called analytic-continental watershed. Analytic philosophy, with its preference for preciseness and narrowing down concepts, geographically is said to refer to the Anglo American world, while continental philosophy engenders its inclination toward an ongoing interpretation and broadening the horizon.

According to Vegard Fusche Moe (2014), however, this distinction is "very limited if not inaccurate" (53), since both originate from the same European philosophical tradition, notably Kant's already mentioned "modern" transcendental philosophy. In Kant's philosophy the term transcendental refers to *a priori* (nonanalytic) elements or judgments which according to him are inevitably entangled in our empirical experience. Transcendental has nothing to do with the usual spiritual connotation of "transcendence," but with the intuitive idea that we cannot know "the pure things" (*Sachen an sich selbst*) without preconceived categories. Fusche Moe furthermore concludes that many philosophers living in mainland Europe are dedicated to the analytic case, while quite a few North American philosophers openly confess to continental philosophy:

> So, in the modern world, geography indicates little about philosophical preferences. . . . AP [analytical philosophy, rw] has shared the problem-oriented and scientific-empirical outlook of the natural sciences, that is, its focus is to search for knowledge and truth in a rationalistic framework where a problem becomes divided and reduced into its smaller parts, analysed and explained in terms of logic or by the laws of nature. On the other hand, CP [continental philosophy, rw] has been concerned with the understanding what appears to be meaningful

for a person in the sense that it has tried to comprehend life as it is lived from the first person point of view. (Fusche Moe 2014, 53)

Although recognizing the blurring limits between the precise and the long-winded and subjective, I would claim that philosophy of sport still is preoccupied with the Suitsian idea of sport as the voluntary and playful attempt to overcome unnecessary obstacles, with a (often hidden) preference for the (supposed autotelic) amateur-stance. This lusory attitude seems not very appropriate for the case in hand though: endurance sport. Although moments or even periods of a sense of lightness, flow, and pleasure may occur, these sports of long breath are, above all, a matter of monotonous repetition and perseverance rather than joyful, unconcerned play. These stamina sports are about enduring life in the long run with an occasional glimpse of unveiled truth, rather than experiencing a total immersion in un-committal joy. I argue that Sloterdijk's ascetological findings are of utmost importance to fully assess the deeper meaning of endurance sport.

## FROM CYNIC TO KYNIC

Before entering Sloterdijk's *You Must Change Your Life* in more detail we should have a look at his critical but constructive basic attitude toward urgent societal issues in times of secularization and fragmentation. In his *Critique of Cynical Reason* (1987)—his European breakthrough as a public philosopher—Sloterdijk already sighed that contemporary philosophy is in deep agony:

> Faced with its demise, it would like now to be honest and reveal its last secret. It confesses: The great themes, they were evasions and half-truths. Those futile, beautiful, soaring flights—God, Universe, Theory, Praxis, Subject, Object, Body, Spirit, Meaning, Nothingness—all that is nothing. They are nouns for young people, outsiders, clerics, sociologists. (xxvi)

More specifically, Sloterdijk criticizes contemporary societal cynicism. According to him this is a defeatist strategy that inoculates itself for critical resistance, and thus is a case of "enlightened false consciousness" (Sloterdijk 1987, 19). To counter this widespread negativism Sloterdijk calls for a more authentic, thriving and "doggish" cynicism (*kynos* means "dog" in ancient Greek), as exemplified in the lifestyle of the ancient "kynic" Diogenes of Synope. This was a down-to-earth philosopher who lived in a water barrel on the Athens market square, and famously asked Alexander the Great to step out of his way because he obscured the daylight.

Under the heading *In Search of Lost Cheekiness*, Sloterdijk reveals the constructive undercurrent of a plain but philosophical life lived in happy refusal: enlightenment through unmasking. This results in what I would coin a tactile post-transcendental philosophical style. (Which however largely lacks William James' vein for seeking "truth in consequences," which will be treated later on.):

> Ethical living may be good, but naturalness is good too. That is all kynical scandal says. . . . Here begins a laughter containing philosophical truth, which we must call to mind again if only because today everything is bent on making us forget how to laugh. (Sloterdijk 1987, 106)

In his much-debated essay *Rules for the Human Zoo: A Response to the Letter on Humanism*[4] (2009), Sloterdijk nevertheless seems to have become somewhat defeatist, if not cynical in the loathed modern sense. He contends that since the humanizing effect of wise books appears to have expired we should consider more deliberate means to ensure the preservation of Aristotle's characterization of man as a *zoon politikon,* a political animal.

Although Sloterdijk certainly plays around with uncomfortable ideas and controversial issues (e.g., eugenics), I would still argue that his open ended essay also can be interpreted as an ultimate, be it somewhat desperate attempt to revitalize the humanizing power of the written word. Two thousand years after Plato, according to Sloterdijk, wisdom has become obsolete:

> What is left to us in the place of the wise is their writings, in their glinting brilliance and their increasing obscurity. . . . Letters that are not mailed cease to be missives for possible friends: they turn into archived things. . . . Perhaps it occasionally happens that in such researches in the dead cellars of culture the long-ignored texts begin to glimmer, as if distant light flickers over them. Can the archives also come into the Clearing?[5] Everything suggests that archivists have become the successors of the humanists. For the few who still peer around in those archives, the realization is dawning that our lives are the confused answer to questions we were asked in places we have forgotten. (Sloterdijk 2009, 27)

## AN ASCETIC PLANET

In *You Must Change Your Life—On Anthropotechnics* (2013), Sloterdijk has overcome his defeatist position of the *Rules for the Human Zoo* and regained his before-mentioned positive "kynic" attitude. He now frankly explores the idea of man as a natural born training animal, from hunger artists and armless violin players to modern super-athletes and dabbling amateurs. The main title of the book is derived from the *Archaic Torso of Apollo,* the opening sonnet of Rainer Maria Rilke's cycle *New Poems: The Other Part* (1908). During

1905 and 1906, Rilke assisted the famous French sculptor Auguste Rodin as a private secretary. Not knowing how to find poetical inspiration again, Rilke, who suffered from a slender physique and poor health, asks for advice from his admired athletic and virile temporary employer, whose famous, at first sight contemplative statue *The Thinker* at a closer look is a paragon of muscularity, if not of an "explosive nature" (Zwart 2010, 73). Rodin advises the melancholic Rilke to go out, look around and simply produce, write, re-write and so gradually improve his suppressed poetic skills. The determined sculptor suggests the undecided poet to visit museums and zoos, to observe concrete *things*. Life is about activation. Works, first and foremost! If you do not succeed the first time, then simply start anew! The analogy with endurance sport is obvious: training, first and foremost.

In the chapter *Command from the Stone*, Sloterdijk reasons that Rilke's point is not that the statue is a petrified echo only interesting for those who are initiated in ancient Greece, the "humanistically educated." The stone-clog is rather a thing-construct that still sends out an urging appeal to all of us: it takes quite an effort to become a full-blown member of the "planet of the practicing." Referring to Nietzsche's *Thus Spoke Zarathustra* (Nietzsche 2005, 60), Sloterdijk (2013) circularly states that "practice is defined here as any operation that provides or improves the actor's qualification for the next performance of the same operation, whether it is declared as a practice or not" (4). We should therefore learn to revalue training as such, and not just as a means to ends: fitness, health, appearance, prestige, power.

In everyday speech, "ascetic" has the connotation of medieval retreatment in monasteries, but the word originally refers to the Greek *askesis*, which means "practice." For Sloterdijk asceticism represents a wide range of subsequent historical manifestations of striving for excellence through dedicated and meticulously performed training practices. All things considered, our "planet of the practicing" is inhabited by individuals who are constantly and relentlessly training themselves, varying from Stoics, Cynics (Kynics!), and monks to cripples and modern Olympic sport professionals.

Asceticism usually is rather self-focused. These subsequent preferred training regimens may lead to a personal *metanoia*, a turning point, radical reform, or personal mitigation. This might entail trying a different approach, becoming less consumptive, more active, getting fit. The indomitable urge to push ourselves ideally also has a broader societal scope, however. Since planet earth is at the brink of ecological doom we should train ourselves to become better citizens, contributing to a just and sustainable society, Sloterdijk insists. In order to achieve this beckoning perspective of global amelioration we have to change our lives and strive for a new horizon of universal co-operative training practices, or a "general ascetology."

On a collective level this might even result in a literal "renaissance," a rebirth which in Sloterdijk's exuberant philosophical grammar is not bound to fourteenth-century Italy but marks a broader variety of massive societal-ideological turnovers. Since Pierre de Coubertin's introduction of the modern Olympics in 1896 the athletic ideal—so predominant in classic Greek culture, drenched with *agon* (combativeness, rivalry, competiveness) and the importance of physical *askesis*—is in the lead again: "[A] transformation best described as a re-somatisation or a de-spiritualisation of asceticisms" (Sloterdijk 2013, 27).

Sloterdijk furthermore insists that the analogy between forms of sport and forms of discourse and knowledge must be taken as literally as possible. This reintroduction of the powerful body however does not mean that the rational and sensitive soul is put aside. *Physis* and *psyche* are two sides of a coin in the modern athlete: "The completion of the renaissance through the return of the athlete around 1900 encompasses the return of the wise man: in the *panathlon* of intelligence, he makes his own contribution to clarifying the form in which that renaissance continues today" (Sloterdijk 2013, 155).

This inborn striving for betterment can be vented by means of "tension procedures." This is also exemplified in the motto of the modern Olympics: *citius, altius, fortius,* always trying to run faster, to jump higher, and to become stronger: "By producing new configurations between contemplation and fitness, the current 'renaissance' enables new festivals on the plateau of the mountain of improbabilities" (Sloterdijk 2013, 155).

The quintessential point of this inexhaustible human potential for overcoming supposed limits is that we at first have to become fully aware of our ascetic disposition as such. Only those who practice for the sake of practicing are able to finally change their life. So, paradoxically, only an autotelic basic attitude may lead to heterotelic results: a personal *metanoia* or a collective renaissance:

> For the primal ethical imperative 'You must change your life!' to be followed, therefore, it is initially necessary for the practising to become aware of their exercises as exercises, that is to say as forms of life that engage the practising person. The reason for this is self-evident: if the players are themselves inescapably affected by what they play and how they play it (and how it has been drilled into them to play it), they will only have access to the bridge of their self-change by recognizing the games in which they are entangled for what they are. (Sloterdijk 2013, 145)

The tension between training programs as such and their implicit transformative power prompts Sloterdijk to refute Wittgenstein's statement that trying to define sport and games are just "language games." He argues that

Wittgenstein may be right when he argues that the meaning of a word is determined by its real usage. What he seems to miss, however, is that the decisive factor is the refinement of that usage through ardent training practices. If once internalized and engrained, asceticism implies freedom and a high potential for change: "This supposed end in itself is, in truth, the medium in which the conversion of possessed rule-applications to free exercises take place" (Sloterdijk 2013, 145).

In sum, for Sloterdijk ascetic practices, though potential mediators, are never sheer means to straightforward hedonistic ends. Shallow ends include such as in the vicinity of mass-sport often used buzz-words as "interaction," "communication," "health," and the "enhancement industry," with its uncanny "departments of plastic surgery, fitness management, wellness service and systemic doping" (Sloterdijk 2013, 338). Well-performed and well-understood practices must also touch upon something essential that we have lost on our way to *homo compensator* in technotopia[6]: understanding that life has more of a Sisyphean effort to get a glimpse of unconcealed being than being a one-dimensional tailor-made training program that linearly leads to personal growth. This is why so many natural born practitioners are still inclined to invest so much energy in initially frustrating practices. Putting in a lot of at first sight futile effort may lead to a sudden breakthrough of facility, Sloterdijk (2013) argues:

> All somewhat advanced civilizations make use of the observation that every active person is dyed in the lye of their activities until the miracle of "second nature" takes place and they perform the near-impossible almost effortlessly. The highest theorem of explicit training theories, then, is that ability subjected to persistent furthering tension produces, almost "of its own accord", heightened ability. (321)

## DIALOGIC MIRRORING AND CONSEQUENTIAL TRUTH

As will have become clear by now, Sloterdijk's meandering philosophical style is continental rather than analytical. He is ever searching for deeper meaning and understanding and broadening perspectives rather than striving "for clear-cut objective explanation, logic, rigidity, conceptual clarity and narrowing down concepts" (Fusche Moe 2014, 53).

In order to comprehend life at large better, Sloterdijk calls for daring readings of all sort of narratives, from canonic to common. He therefore explicitly confesses to hermeneutics, the philosophical art of interpretation that is so prominently present in his guides Nietzsche and Heidegger. Provocative and challenging interpretations have a decisive advantage over obedient close-readings, Sloterdijk (1987) contends: "Others often really do perceive things about me that escape my attention and conversely. They possess the advantage of distance, which I can profit from only retrospectively through dialogic mirroring" (19).

For Sloterdijk, "author" refers to a wide range of interpretations. In order to get a broader perspective on his stakes, he skillfully oscillates between peer-reviewed scientific writings, literature, pulp fiction, and un-canonical anecdotal reports of the fringes of society. This broad-band dialogic mirroring style in *You Must Change Your Life* indeed results in strengthening the central hypothesis of human life as a series of practices gradually brought to perfection, ranging from illustrating bibles to cycling up the steepest of climbs.

For the sake of "objectivity," and in order to avoid a vicious cycle in which every explanation circularly refers to another, classical hermeneutics attempts to exchange weaker interpretations for stronger ones in a more or less linear way. Twentieth-century thinkers like Paul Ricoeur, Martin Heidegger, and Hans-Georg Gadamer are less denunciative of circularity in reasoning, since interpretive recurrence is almost unavoidable. Sloterdijk picks the best of both worlds and introduces the idea of a *circulus virtuosos*; a virtuous circle which denotes a complex chain of events that reinforce themselves through a feedback loop with a favorable result—upwardly oriented spiralism or vertical tension, one might say. Sloterdijk (2013) contends, "Through exact descriptions of the *circulus virtuosos*, it becomes explicable how accomplishment leads to higher accomplishment and success to expanded success" (321).

Sloterdijk (2013) stresses the importance of changing our lives into a more ecological direction: "I am to develop into a fakir of coexistence with everyone and everything, and reduce my footprint in the environment to the trail of a feather" (449). In the last paragraphs of *You Must Change Your Life* he also refers to a societal tool which might help to realize the ecological renaissance on the collective level:

> Although communism was a conglomeration of a few correct ideas and many wrong ones, its reasonable part—the understanding that shared life interests of the highest order can only be realized within a horizon of co-operative asceticisms—will have to assert itself anew sooner or later. It presses for a macrostructure of global immunizations: co-immunism. Civilization is one such structure. Its monastic rules must be drawn up now or never; they will encode the forms of anthropotechnics that befit existence in the context of all contexts. Wanting to live by them would mean making a decision: to take on the good habits of shared survival in daily exercises. (Sloterdijk 2013, 451–452)

## INTO THE PRAGMATIC MOOD

Classic pragmatism, with its predilection for functionalism and consequentialism, may help to concretize Sloterdijk's "metanoetical" and "renaissancistic" message of taking on the good habits of shared survival in daily exercises. William James (1842–1910), one of the founding fathers of pragmatism, contends that there is no transcendental "truth" but nothing but a "reality" that efficiently has to be dealt with. He also coined the idea of "truth in consequences": when different approaches lead to the same desirable result, both are true. It should be noted, however, that James' probably best-turned phrases "truth's cash value" (1907a, 200) and "the true is only the expedient in our way of thinking" (222) often are used out of context. Their meaning is far more subtle than bluntly stating that any idea with some practical utility is true. James' pragmatic ponderings closely resemble Sloterdijk's process-oriented ideas on asceticism. James stresses the importance of the *process* from beliefs—or "thoughts in rest" (1901/1902, 293)—to true actions. (In our case, this means switching over from Rilke's passive melancholic mood to Rodin's active athleticism.)

Sloterdijk briefly refers to James' idea that conversions may also happen in a "sick soul" or a "divided self," even "without any religious turn" (2013, 306). He also pays credit to the nineteenth-century pragmatist conviction that the self-production of humans "is made explicit via study of the *vita activa*" (320). And, finally, he also mentions the "piecemeal supranaturalism" which "perfectly suited the pragmatic immanentism of the Modern Age" (371), both put forward in James' *The Varieties of Religious Experience*.

The relation between Sloterdijk's post-transcendental hermeneutic continentalism with a touch of moralism and the pedagogic vein in James' interpretive pragmatism is more intricate, however. First, one should note the striking similarity between Sloterdijk's idea that a "persistent furthering tension produces, almost 'of its own accord,' heightened ability" (321) and James' ponderings in *The Energies of Man* on the benefits of a second wind (or "second breath" as the Dutch saying goes), which may accrue to us when we push ourselves to (and over) our limits:

> But if an unusual necessity forces us to press onward, a surprising thing occurs. The fatigue gets worse up to a certain critical point, when gradually or suddenly it passes away, and we are fresher than before. We have evidently tapped a level of new energy, masked until then by the fatigue-obstacle usually obeyed. There may be layer after layer of this experience. A third and a fourth "wind" may supervene. (James 1907b, 7)

Also, James' idea of conversions—either religious or profane—imply the possibility for relieving one's vertical tension through striving for a "personal best." Evidently humans are prone to save their own skin in the vortex of being. But at the same time our arduous training practices may imply a sense of modesty. Also, James acknowledges that a personal optimum often is the best we can get: "[W]hen we touch our own upper limit and live in our own highest center of energy, we may call ourselves saved, no matter how much higher someone else's centre may be" (James 1901/1902, 165). Sloterdijk even completely strips conversions from their religious connotations. Changing your life is a matter of getting on your feet and practicing like hell:

> The whole complex known as ethics comes from the gesture of conversion to ability. Conversion is not the transition from one belief system to another; the original conversion takes place as an exit from the passivist mode of existence in coincidence with the entrance into the activist mode. It is the nature of the matter that this activation and the avowal of the practising life comes to the same thing. (Sloterdijk 2013, 195)

When we dialogically and consequentially reconsider the given that today humans are natural born athletic ascetics with a vertical tension that has somehow to be vented, we can nothing but conclude that seriously practiced endurance sport is an involuntary attempt (to turn Suits' before-mentioned phrase of game-playing as the voluntary attempt to overcome unnecessary obstacles) to overcome a necessary obstacle toward a meaningful and enduring life.

Still, the official philosophy of sport usually concentrates on jolliness. In *Agon in Nietzsche,* Yunus Tuncel (2013) reminds us of the fierce roots of competitive physicality, however: "With the ancient Greeks, the agonal spirit had already existed in poetry, mythology, arts, and *athletics* (italics mine), before it re-produced itself in thought with the rise of philosophy" (255). In the same period during which Rilke became re-inspired by an archaic torso with a six-pack, Nietzsche feverishly attempted to revitalize this ancient spirit in order to unmask the feebleness of his own era. Over a century later Tuncel (2013) sighs that "agonal feelings do not have a sufficient, wider acceptance today, sometimes not even among the competing forces" (257). Nietzsche's ideal of a strong agonistic individualism has been reduced to the playful "demands of the populace for self-preservation, for mundane affairs, for sameness and equality; monolithicity rules. . . . What counts is the excitement of the masses, a petty spectacle of scoring goals" (Tuncel, 2013, 257).

By performing "agonal" contests on the razor's edge sport nevertheless still can be a powerful means to a serious end: seeking unpolished knowledge, cultivating virtue, and enhancing the good life. This means fully opting for the challenging life William James argued for after experiencing a numbing complacency during a conference at a peaceful oasis for scholarly retreatment in upstate New York:

At Chautauqua, there were no racks, even in the place's historical museum; and no sweat, except possibly the gentle moisture on the brow of some lecturer, or on the sides of some player in the ball-field. . . . It looks indeed, thought I, as if the romantic idealists with their pessimism about our civilization were, after all, quite right. An irremediable flatness is coming over the world. . . . The higher heroisms and the old rare flavors are passing out of life. (James 1899, 6)

## INTO THE STRENUOUS MOOD

In *The Heights of Humanity: Endurance Sport and the Strenuous Mood*, Hochstetler and Hopsicker (2012) pick up the plea for high spirits and matching physics by arguing that endurance sports have special benefits to offer when it comes to fighting flatness. For them there is a fundamental difference between occasional joggers and riders ("breadth") and dedicated runners and cyclists ("depth"). They argue that the classic philosophical pragmatism of William James and John Dewey is the key to understand why these sports can make life significant and worthwhile. Strenuously practiced endurance sport opens the possibilities for "recovering humanity" in a manner qualitatively different from the "transcendental approach" toward sport as distracting from everyday dullness (Hochstetler and Hopsicker 2012, 118).

This specific brand of "transcendentalism" Hochstetler and Hopsicker refer to has been developed in the later 1820s and 1830s in the United States. Building on Immanuel Kant's already mentioned idea of "transcendentals" as intuitive but necessary conditions for knowledge, representatives such as Ralph Waldo Emerson and Henry David Thoreau rather rely on (transcendental) subjective intuition rather than the rigid empiricism of the pragmatists.

Hochstetler and Hopsicker agree with Anderson's (2001) transcendentalist line of thought that anyone who leisurely and occasionally participates in sport applies for the possibility of "growth through commitment." They contend, however, that only those who are truly dedicated to the endurance case have a higher potential for personal growth: "Because of their engagement, these athletes have a *heightened* chance of meeting possibility, a *heightened* chance of establishing creativity, and a *heightened* chance of learning about self" (Hochstetler & Hopsicker 2012, 120). To substantiate their claims they work up the idea of a process oriented "increased ownership" for serious practitioners who consider sport more than an appropriate tool for temporary "distancing" themselves from the daily drag. True dedication and serious suffering are favorable tools for creating a meaningful life through trying to improve one's personal best:

> Both the jogger and runner may find their respective movement outlets enticing as a way to combat the restlessness of routine life. However, the runner

even has more reason to anticipate movement and endurance sport, not only as a respite from the work world but also in the recognition that through these efforts one gradually develops an identity as an endurance athlete. (Hochstetler & Hopsicker 2012, 121)

Other than ball games, sprinting and all sports that require highly developed motor skills, endurance sports also have special benefits to offer for the ageing athlete: "many runners and cyclists can achieve their personal best times during their 30s and even their 40s" (Hochstetler & Hopsicker 2012, 121). There is, however, a downside to dedication and patience, carved in the sporting subject over decades of training, the authors rightly argue. Whereas youth normally comes with agility, joy, and freedom from worry, coming of age implies less flexible limbs, and more need of physical care, practical wisdom, moderation, punctuality, meticulous devotion and abstinence of all sorts, and therefore the danger of living the life of a monomaniac: "It is certainly true that sport can become mechanistic, and on occasion a setting where individual agency becomes squelched" (Hochstetler & Hopsicker 2012, 122).

The pitfall of narrowing down life to asceticism only does not mean however, that endurance sport is dull routine *per se*. There is still an openness for creating a certain distance to the daily drag in the strenuous mood. A life fully lived in training programs still "has the potential to produce deeply meaningful experiences for those athletes called to sporting practices" (Hochstetler & Hopsicker 2012, 122). Those who are able to endure life in the strenuous mood have a unique chance to "drive life into a corner." Hochstetler and Hopsicker (2012) contend, "While these qualities are available to the weekend warrior, we contend that physical activity, conducted in the strenuous vein, is a fertile ground for experiencing the depth of our humanity" (132).

## POTENTIAL PERILS

In *Normative Concerns for Endurance Athletes* (2016), Hochstetler and Hopsicker somewhat tone down their potent pragmatist plea for the strenuous mood. Now they argue in favor of a more holistically oriented attempt to fulfill Aristotle's notion of *eudaimonia*, or human flourishing, the final goal in his virtue ethics. Other than gasping joggers, somewhat corpulent weekend warriors and easygoing breaststroke swimmers, long distance runners, serious cyclists and smooth crawlers namely may face a "potential dark side" of their hyper-focused training programs. By becoming glassy slaves of the repetitive rhythm of absolving daily mileages and personalized training programs, the truly dedicated ones are prone to neglect their social environment. Frenetic fanatics may "relinquish other interests in pursuit of excellence in their particular sport" (Hochstetler & Hopsicker 2016, 1). Say the potential perils of damaged interpersonal relations and marital problems: "To avoid becoming either a minion or puny fellow, one must find some way to navigate the various tensions inherent with endurance sport participation" (Hochstetler & Hopsicker 2016, 13).

In the same eudaimonistic vein Gunnar Breivik (2010) has argued for putting the all too strenuous sporty mood into perspective. He suggests well-roundedness and concentration as alternatives for theories that strive for excellence: "perfection is an attractive choice but no obligation" (87). The idea of a well-balanced Golden Mean—say between recklessness and cowardice—is prominent in Aristotle's virtue ethics. Notably the notion of *phronēsis*, or practical wisdom, is appropriate for the case at hand: how much strenuousness can we endure in our search for the good life? It should be reminded, however, that, somewhat similar to Sloterdijk and James, Aristotle in his *Nicomachean Ethics* opts for an excellence-oriented agonistic approach in sport:

> And as in the Olympic Games it is not the most beautiful and strongest that are crowned but those who compete (for it is some of these that are victorious), so those who act win, and rightly win, the noble and good things in life. (Aristotle 1999, 13)

Trying to win, getting the best out of yourself, pushing yourself to your limits is not just a matter of narcissism, it also refers to the intrinsic value of the strenuous life. Besides the danger of social isolation, Hochstetler and Hopsicker (2016) warn of the possibility for endurance athletes to develop the well-known overtraining syndrome. In addition, Sloterdijk (2013) acknowledges the perils of living the strenuous life close to or sometimes even over the edge. Still, the positive effects of super-compensation after extreme training sessions prevail if well-performed:

> The rhythms of regeneration hold the secret of the overexertion that leads to higher performance levels. This phenomenon has been intuitively comprehensible since time immemorial, and had already been exploited for intensive training session in antiquity; on the other hand, the ancients were also familiar with the phenomena of overtraining that appear if regeneration rhythms had been disregarded. (320–321)

Train hard, rest hard. The strenuous life is about learning to know thyself.

## CYCLING UPHILL AT YOUR OWN PACE

The distinctive advantage of endurance sports as a preferential mold for venting our ascetic tendencies is that these are within reach of the masses. Elite runners, cyclists, and triathletes of course have special talents that are beyond the reach of mortals. But those who are willing to spend sufficient training hours and develop stamina may also enter the Hall of Fame of long distance race finishers, or perhaps even become age-group winners. Here again the overarching adage is try hard to get the best out of your very self, rather than overtaking opponents or winning a specific contest. As triathlon-trainer Tim Heming (2015) argues:

> All of us, whatever level we are, aim to race faster, higher and stronger.... The breadth and depth of triathlon experience can be truly exceptional.... Don't get caught up in others' targets. Instead, create your own triathlon journey and remember to enjoy it. (78–79)

Of course, one may decry an occasional smile on a competitor's face during a long distance endurance event. My quite educated guess however is that triathletes, or endurance aficionados at large, enjoy their sport in a far more modest manner than, say, soccer- or basketball-players, with their vehement outbursts in the petty spectacle of scoring goals. The stealthy smile of an endurance athlete is an accidental belch drenched in a sea of indefatigable resilience.

Precisely this orientation on acquired stamina rather than innate talent makes endurance sport easier to perform than say soccer or gymnastics. Notably cycling has special benefits to offer for the crowd. The noble art of pedaling exerts a relatively low impact on the limbs, and does not require highly developed motor skills. In the seventies, the Dutch cyclist Joop Zoetemelk was not even able to absolve a very elementary obstacle-run during a TV-show, nor was he able to pull himself up at the horizontal bar. Still he won the Tour de France in 1980.

On top of it, widely practiced cycling has more than just a sporty potency. It might help us move toward a more sustainable lifestyle. Hopping on a bike more often certainly would make the world a better place. The Danish philosophical cyclist Steen Nepper Larsen picks up Sloterdijk's slumbering ascetic-metanoetic message and paves the way for a massive strenuous cycling philosophy for the better. He argues that in contrast to a modern sports utility vehicle, a bicycle is the perfect contemporary "anthropotechnical" extension piece of the human body: "Relatively primitive bike technology fosters an *ecstatic-present-attentive* being. One might say that I become bigger than my own flesh" (Nepper Larsen 2010, 30). Once you have experienced the possibility of overcoming yourself on two un-motorized wheels there is no way back. Mountains are not to be messed with. Either you climb them or you leave them alone. But once you are sufficiently trained they keep winking: "Emanating from the mountains of the world, a vertical imperative hits the horizontal human. Pull yourself together, leave the lowlands and conquer the summit!" (Nepper Larsen 2010, 30).

Creating your very own upwardly oriented challenge, following the commandment from the stone to elevate yourself definitely has more potential for depth than unconcernedly pedaling or jogging along. Really pushing yourself to your limits will quite probably indeed result in Hochstetler's and Hopsicker's heightened chances of learning about self through tough stages of "increased ownership." Even more, once infected with the endurance virus, even somewhat puny fellows as Joop Zoetemelk ostensibly may become dedicated minions of the better sort.

When it comes to actual improvement of our lives in Sloterdijk's renaissancistic perspective, we should keep in mind, however, that competitive sport, even in its mildest manifestations, to a certain degree is also always about fight, which is the very metaphor for our, regarding the inconvenient truth we are facing, literally unsustainable lifestyle. But as Sloterdijk stresses: for every result-driven professional there are a thousand well-willing amateurs. Properly performed endurance sport nevertheless can help to overcome the tension between competitiveness and coexistence. By revaluing the concept of *askesis* as a contemporary and relatively clean and green means to fight the struggle with and against oneself, we may overcome the uncompromising fight against our natural environment and transform the human condition into a coexistent agony with the world (Welters, 2014).

Nevertheless, we should avoid using endurance sport as a straightforward mean to an in itself praiseworthy end. There should always remain a nucleus of indeterminateness in our congenital tendency for asceticism, beyond the idea of linear growth toward a better and fuller self, and in the long run perhaps even a better world. True asceticism is not about using proper means to straightforward ends, Sloterdijk (2013) argues. It is rather about learning to endure life as such:

> But if man genuinely produces man, it is precisely not work and its concrete results, not even the "work on oneself" so widely praised in recent times, let alone through the alternatively invoked phenomena of "interaction" or "communication": it is through life in forms of practice. Practice is defined here as any operation that provides or improves the actor's qualification for the next performance of the same operation, whether it is declared as a practice or not. (4)

In a similar vein James (1907b) underlines the already mentioned beneficial experience of a second wind, which also helps to improve every next performance of the same operation, so that the "higher heroisms and the old rare flavors" (6) just will not pass out of life. To counter the flatness that indisputably is coming over the world we should put ourselves on the rack, not just every now and then but on a basis as regular as possible.

In conclusion, the net sum of the preceding encounter of continentalism and pragmatism is that we are all natural born ascetics in a world filled with hindrances. Since they learn to endure life with all its defects, those who learn to really agonize themselves in order to optimize their ascetic potentialities will become better humans in the end. Strenuously performed sports that take long breath—competitive or not—are a preferential tool for carving out some idea of enduring meaning. This easily accessible but meanwhile Sisyphean form of asceticism should be performed in the great wide and preferably mountainous open. Only there we can escape the daily grind of the horizontal life. Rather on your own or in small group, fairly ahead of the pack and the peloton.

By revaluing the Sisyphean concept of *askesis* as a contemporary and relatively clean and green means to fight the struggle with and against oneself, we may overcome the uncompromising fight against our natural environment and transform the human condition into a "coexistent agony" with the world. This, however, without throwing the competitive, proto-agonistic baby that still lingers in us out with the bathwater:

> Perhaps agonism is not a sufficient response to all human suffering; however, it is one response. Just like the tragic human, it accepts human suffering at least in two areas; it channels cruelty and destruction unto culturally accepted arenas and it enables humans to deal with loss and death. It must also be mentioned that agonism promotes strong individuality, the best response to human suffering. (Tuncel 2013, 256–57)

All things considered, only the physically seasoned life is worth to be lived. To turn Bernard Suits' gratuitous definition of game-playing around: In a meaningful life, endurance sport is an involuntary attempt to overcome necessary obstacles.

## NOTES

1. A more comprehensive academic version of this chapter can be found in:
   Welters, R., Towards a Sustainable Philosophy of Endurance
Sport: Cycling for Life. Springer, Library of Ethics & Applied Philosophy 37, 2019. This book deals with the wider philosophical implications of endurance sport and eco-philosophy.

2. Kant made a shift from classical metaphysics to the idea that the human experience implies a fundamentally subject-based component, instead of being an activity that directly comprehends the things as they are in themselves. In shorthand: "transcendentals" are intuitive but necessary conditions for acquiring knowledge of what is usually referred to as "the world."

3. The following analysis of Sloterdijk's ideas on human practicing is based on Welters (2016).

4. This refers to Martin Heidegger's *Letter on Humanism* (1949).

5. The place where according truth can be revealed (*aletheia*), an idea which has been taken up by Heidegger.

6. Sloterdijk is anything but a dystopian or cynical thinker when it comes to technology. The term "anthropotechnics" in the subtitle *You Must Change Your Life* refers to this optimistic attitude. "Salvation, for Sloterdijk, lies in just the area where Heidegger believed perdition lay: that is, in the realm of technology. Yet technology, for Sloterdijk, seldom has to do with machines. It is mental and spiritual technology that interests him: the techniques with which human beings have historically made themselves secure on the Earth" (Kirsch 2015).

## REFERENCES

Anderson, D. (2001). Recovering Humanity: Movement, Sport and Nature. *Journal of the Philosophy of Sport* 28, 140–150.

Aristotle. (1999). *Ethica Nicomacheia*. Kitchener: Batoche Books.

Breivik, G. (2010). Philosophical Perfectionism—Consequences and Implications for Sport. *Sport, Ethics and Philosophy* 4(1), 87–105.

Fusche Moe, V. (2014). The Philosophy of Sport and Continental Philosophy. In C. Torres (Ed.), *The Bloomsbury Companion to the Philosophy of Sport* (pp. 52–65). London: Bloomsbury.

Gorris, L., & Kurbjuweit, D. (2008). Philosopher Peter Sloterdijk on the Tour de France: "The Riders are Just Regular Employees." *Der Spiegel Online International*. Available at: http://www.spiegel.de/international/eur ope/philosopher-peter-sloterdijk-on-the-tour-de-france-the-riders-are-just-regular-employees-a-565111.html

Heidegger, M. (2008 (1927)). *Being and Time*. New York: Harper & Row.

Heidegger, M. (1949). *Letter on Humanism*. Available at: http://pacificinstitute.org/pdf/Letter_on_%20Humanism.pdf

Heming, T. (2015). *Join the Club*. In 220 Triathlon, March 2015, 78–79.

Hochstetler, D., & Hopsicker, P.M. (2016). Normative Concerns for Endurance Athletes. *Journal of the Philosophy of Sport* 43(3), 335–349.

Hochstetler, D., & Hopsicker, P.M. (2012). The Heights of Humanity: Endurance Sport and the Strenuous Mood. *Journal of the Philosophy of Sport* 39(1), 117–136.

James, W. (1907a). *Pragmatism, A New Name for Some Old Ways of Thinking, Popular Lectures on Philosophy*. New York: Longmans, Green, & Co.

James, W. (1907b). *The Energies of Man*. The American Magazine (reprint). Available at: https://archive.org/stream/energiesofmen00jameuoft/energiesofmen00jameuoft_djvu.txt

James, W. (1901/ 1902). *The Varieties of Religious Experience. A Study in Human Nature*. Available at: https://worldu.edu/library/william_james_var.pdf

James, W. (1899). *What Makes a Life Significant?* Available at: http://philosophy.lander.edu/intro/articles/jameslife-a.pdf

Kahn, J. (2009). *Divine Discontent: The Religious Imagination of W. E. B. Du Bois*. Oxford: Oxford University press.

Krajeweski, B. (1989). Critique of Cynical Reason, Peter Sloterdijk. *The Journal of the Midwest Modern Language Association* 22(1), 61–64.

Kretchmar, R.S. (1982). '"Distancing:" An Essay on Abstract Thinking in Sport Performances. *Journal of the Philosophy of Sport* 9, 6–18.

Kretchmar, R.S. (1975). From Test to Contest: An Analysis of Two Kinds of Counterpoint in Sport. *Journal of the Philosophy of Sport* II, 23–30.

Nepper Larsen, S. (2010). Becoming a Cyclist—Phenomenological Reflections on Cycling. In J. Ilundáin-Agurruza and M.W. Austin (Eds.), *Cycling Philosophy for Everyone: A Philosophical Tour de Force* (pp. 27–39). Chichester: Wiley Blackwell.

Reid, H.L. (2009). Sport, Philosophy, and the Quest for Knowledge. *Journal of the Philosophy of Sport* 36(1), 40–49.

Sloterdijk, P. (2013/2009). *You Must Change Your Life—On Anthropotechnics*. Cambridge: Malden.

Sloterdijk, P. (2009/1999). Rules for the Human Zoo. A Response to the *Letter on Humanism. Environment and Planning D: Society and Space* 27, 12–28. Available at: https://rekveld.home.xs4all.nl/tech/Sloterdijk_RulesForTheHumanZoo.pdf

Sloterdijk, P. (1987/1983). *Critique of Cynical Reason*. Minneapolis: University of Minnesota Press.

Suits, B. (2005/1978). *The Grasshopper: Games, Life, and Utopia*. Ontario: Broadview Press.

Suits, B. (1988). Tricky Triad: Games, Play, and Sport. *Journal of the Philosophy of Sport* 15, 1–9.

Tuncel, Y. (2013). *Agon in Nietzsche*. Milwaukee: Marquette University Press.

Wittgenstein, L. (1978/1953). *Philosophical Investigations*. London: Blackwell.

Welters, R. (2016). On ascetic Practices and Hermeneutical Cycles. *Sport, Ethics and Philosophy* 10(4), 430–443. doi:10.1080/17511321.2016.1201526.

Welters, R. (2014). Sport and the Environment—Ecosophical and Metanoetical Intersections. In C. Torres (Ed.), *The Bloomsbury companion to the Philosophy of Sport* (pp. 163–179). London: Bloomsbury.

Zwart, H. (2010). Wordt ons Leven Anders? Over Genomics en Zelfarbeid—Beschouwingen naar Aanleiding van Peter Sloterdijks *Du musst dein Leben ändern. Tijdschrift voor Gezondheidszorg en Ethiek* 2(20), 73–76.

*Chapter 3*

# Floyd Landis, Endurance Sport, and the Aesthetics of Tension

Tim Elcombe

On July 20, 2006, American cyclist Floyd Landis launched a brazen solo attack against the peloton near the start of Stage 17 of the *Tour de France*. A prerace favorite with the temporary retirement of Lance Armstrong and the absence of other top cyclists involved in a Spanish government doping probe, Landis entered the final mountain stage of *La Tour* in eleventh place. The race leader at the start of Stage 16, Landis experienced a disastrous final climb on July 19 and fell far behind the leaders in the overall standings. With only four stages remaining, Landis' chances at wearing yellow in the shadow of the Champs-Élysées in Paris seemed hopeless. But, incredibly, one day later during Stage 17 Landis rode away from the rest of the main field for over 120 km to decisively claim the stage and move to third overall. Only 30 seconds behind leader Oscar Pereiro following his monumental stage win, Landis' superior time trialing skill propelled him into the yellow jersey at the end of Stage 19, ultimately securing victory in the 93rd edition of the *Tour de France*.

Learned and casual observers alike described Landis' Stage 17 performance as perhaps the greatest in the history of stage-race road cycling. However, mere days following the Tour's conclusion, World Anti-Doping Agency (WADA) officials announced that Landis' urine sample collected after his epic ride revealed abnormally high testosterone to epitestosterone ratios—an indication of the use of banned synthetic substances to enhance performance. *Tour de France* officials immediately stripped Landis of his title in lieu of the doping violation, awarding the yellow jersey to second place finisher Pereiro. Landis initially claimed his innocence, unsuccessfully mounting public relations campaigns and legal challenges in an attempt to overturn his disqualification.

Years later we now know Landis, by his own admission, violated performance enhancement rules of cycling; but questions remain as to how we ought to view his Stage 17 victory. Although enhanced through illegal means, Landis still performed a feat few cycling afficionados will forget, against a field of riders that included many who would similarly test positive for or raise suspicions about doping offences at some point in the coming years. With this issue serving as the backdrop, I will explore an implicit (yet central) experiential aspect of endurance sport—the tension between human doing (intentional "actions") and undergoing (receptive "suffering").

It is the appreciation for the complexity of human existence within ever-changing "lifeworlds" (in the language of American philosopher John Dewey) that in part distinguishes the American philosophical—particularly pragmatic—project from more traditional approaches to philosophy. Recognizing the centrality of this pragmatic sense of active tension, I suggest, helps us understand why both participants and spectators are drawn to sport. The tension implicit in human experience between the possible and impossible gives sport its force as a meaningful form of life. As well, this tension between inefficiency and evolution also provides an explanation as to how we set our aesthetic and subsequently our moral and logical compasses in contexts such as endurance sport. Appreciating this pivotal idea, therefore, offers an experientially engaged starting point to pragmatically address many pertinent human issues arising in sport, including the structure of our games and the role technology might best play in athletic competition. But beyond endurance sport, understanding the tension between doing and undergoing (embodied by the story of Floyd Landis) helps us better appreciate key features of American philosophy.

## FLOYD LANDIS: A REAL AMERICAN (IDEOLOGICAL) TALE

The story of Floyd Landis, the person, embodies ideological tenets often associated with (on certain interpretations) the American social experiment. Born in Pennsylvania's Lancaster County, Landis grew up in a strict Mennonite household. Despite his parents' disapproval of television, movies, or dancing, Landis received permission to mountain bike—assuming his legs were covered when riding. When his love of cycling turned to the road, Landis' father attempted to dissuade him from continuing this pursuit by assigning extra chores to soak up the teenager's time and energy. Landis responded by riding in the middle of the night, asserting his individuality and willingness to "do what it takes" to succeed—creating tension between his family's religious beliefs (grounded in America's commitment to religious freedom) and Landis' right to self-expression (Murphy, 2006).

Eventually Landis moved away from the family's Pennsylvania home to craft his own narrative in California, pursuing a career in professional cycling. Embodying the American meritocratic ideal that within each individual the capacity to succeed exists, Landis' talent, efforts, and commitment eventually landed him a contract with Lance Armstrong's dominant U.S. Postal Services team and a place on their *Tour de France* roster. Armstrong and his "American" team took on the world, rolling through the villages and over the mountain passes of France in the biggest and most important cycling Grand Tour. Playing the role of loyal teammate, Landis sacrificed his body and personal aspirations on a daily basis to support an American hero reach heights never before seen in cycling—in a sport previously of little interest to his home nation. Armstrong's force of personality, compelling (and highly public) story of survival from cancer, willingness to push the limits of cycling through the use of technology and tactics, in addition to his sheer physical and psychological power, catapulted him to the top of the podium at the *Tour de France* for seven straight years and captured the imagination of Americans at home. But Armstrong's success depended in large part on the strength of his team, the willingness of talented American riders like George Hincapie, Tyler Hamilton, and Landis to sacrifice their own ambitions to support the greater good (Murphy, 2006).

After three years of *domestique* work for Armstrong's pursuit of glory, Landis flexed his free market muscle and joined the rival Phonak team, eventually becoming the Swiss-based squad's lead general classification rider—the rugged individual at the head of the pack for whom all the others sacrificed. In his first year as team leader, Landis battled the Texan megastar on the road and off. When Armstrong rode off into the sunset (temporarily) following the 2005 season, opportunities for rivals such as Jan Ulrich and Ivan Basso opened up to return the yellow jersey to European shoulders. However, Spanish authorities' *Operation Puerto* doping probe resulted in Ulrich, Basso, and other top contenders' exclusion from the 2006 *Tour de France*. Landis suddenly found himself a favorite to win the race and keep *La Tour* title with an American. With his epic Stage 17 ride defying cycling logic and convention, displaying athletic courage and a willingness to suffer completely to realize his championship ambitions, Landis won the 2006 Tour (temporarily) in an unparalleled display of American exceptionalism (Murphy, 2016; 2006).

In the days following, however, officials stripped Landis of his title based on the urine test results. Landis challenged the findings, claiming innocence and mobilizing a team of lawyers (funded in large part by supporter donations) to overturn the decision. Already forced out of competing post-Tour due to previously scheduled hip surgery, Landis also incurred a two-year cycling ban. After the long hiatus and unsuccessful legal maneuvers, Landis struggled to find a team willing to take him on until he eventually raced in 2009 for a relatively inconsequential American team in hopes of impressing Grand Tour squads. But Landis could not regain his form or spur major team interest, leaving him with only sub-elite team and race opportunities (Murphy, 2016).

Landis felt betrayed by the cycling community, particularly his former squad members, treated as a sacrificial lamb in a sport world enmeshed in quietly accepted doping practices. With his professional frustrations mounting, Landis decided to break cycling's Omerta, the professional peloton's code of silence, and simultaneously revealed to anti-doping officials, race organizers, and the media the inner workings of the sport's culture of rampant doping practices and systematic cover ups. He named names, most notably former teammates Armstrong and Hincapie, while sitting on the sidelines of the 2010 early season primer race, the Tour of California. Despite Armstrong's denials and subsequent character assassinations of Landis, U.S. Department of Justice officials invoked the power of subpoena to impel other racers to corroborate the accusations. Following the controversial decision by Federal prosecutors to eventually drop fraud charges against Armstrong, the United States Anti-Doping Agency (USADA) used the accumulated evidence to continue an investigation into the doping allegations. After three years Armstrong finally succumbed, admitting during a tearful 2013 Oprah interview in the face of overwhelming evidence and a lifetime competition ban that he used a myriad of banned performance enhancing tactics to win his seven *Tour de France* titles. Landis' invocation of his right to free speech through the power of the press ultimately ended his association with professional cycling, and after years of personal struggles he now finds himself as an entrepreneur starting up a recreational cannabis product company in Colorado (Murphy, 2016).

Landis' tale, in all its messiness and complication, is an example of one narrative often weaved about the American ideological project. His story is one of freedom, choice, opportunity, justice, loyalty, ambition, individualism, truth, and courage; but it is also one of failure, temptation, redemption, and acceptance. America's self-image, at least its more "masculine" Rocky Balboa version, embodies these very tenets (cf. Rego, 2009; Yarbrough, 1998): one can find her own way, push to new heights, but may also need to respond in the face of disappointment, loss, and cruelty. The principles wedded to this version of America's national narrative evoke inevitable conflicts between self reliance and community, freedom and commitment, rights and responsibilities, injustice and fairness, power and acquiescence, ambition and acceptance, progress and limits, equality and dessert, past and future.

But, importantly for the purpose of this volume, the story of Floyd Landis serves as more than an opportunity to philosophically reflect on American sociopolitical ideologies. Floyd Landis, particularly through the lens of his Stage 16 and 17 rides at the 2006 *Tour de France*, again plays the role of muse to reveal crucial aspects of American philosophy. In particular, Landis' failings and subsequent response in these two consecutive stages in the French Alps highlight the central role of aesthetics in the writings of classical pragmatists including Charles Peirce, William James, and particularly John Dewey. In turn, the pragmatic emphasis on aesthetics provides us with an experientially thick way to view Landis' Stage 17 performance.

## THE AESTHETICS OF HUMAN "DOING" IN SPORT

For 5 hours, 23 minutes, and 36 seconds on July 20, 2006, Floyd Landis' Stage 17 ride reflected a central reason why humans are attracted to all sports at all levels—the meaningful exhibition (in varying degrees and means) of human "doing." At the conclusion of Stage 15 two days earlier, the first of the three mountain stages scheduled consecutively during the final week of the Tour, Landis rode strongly up the 13.8 kilometers (km) of the famed Alpes d'Huez to regain the yellow jersey he first wore following Stages 11 and 12. Although Landis failed to win at the summit of Alpes d'Huez, his fourth-place stage finish moved him 10 seconds ahead of Pereiro in the cumulative general classification table. Pereiro, however, regained the overall lead the next day at the end of Stage 16 after a strong third place ascent up La Toussuire. Landis, conversely, struggled mightily up the final climb of the day, crossing the line more than 8 minutes behind Pereiro. After enduring two previous days of withering mountain climbs in the French Alps near the end of the brutal three-week Grand Tour race, Landis and his fellow riders then wearily convened at the start line in Saint-Jean-de-Maurienne for the 201 km Stage 17 that included five significant ascents in its course profile.[1]

No longer considered a genuine overall contender after his Stage 16 debacle, the peloton allowed Landis to ride away on the first climb of the day with more than 120 km to traverse before the route's finish. Rather than stay with other breakaway riders for support, Landis rode at a relentless pace and, despite needing to change bikes after breaking a spoke 8 kilometers from the top of the difficult Colombière climb, the Pennsylvanian eventually caught all the riders up the road and dropped any challengers attempting to stay on his wheel. Landis won the stage, nearly 6 minutes ahead of the day's second place rider and more than 7 minutes ahead of Pereiro. Although only third in the general classification at the day's conclusion, his main rivals recognized Landis' epic stage ride made him the overall title favorite with less than a 30-second deficit to overcome in the looming time trial. Sure enough, Landis defeated Pereiro by nearly 90 seconds on the Tour's penultimate day, cementing his victory with only the ceremonial ride into Paris remaining for the general classification contenders.

At home the morning of Stage 17, my wife and I sat riveted by Landis' audacious attempt to reassert himself as a relevant factor in the 2006 Tour. As Landis continued to open the gap on his main competitors and track down breakaway riders still in front of him, our plans to head to work in the morning went by the wayside. Landis astounded many that day, riding what one commentator described "a miracle ride, the most exciting Tour stage—hell, the most amazing bike race—I've ever witnessed" (Lai, 2006). The *Cycling News* (2006) described Landis' ride as "without a shadow of a doubt ... one of the finest stages in modern *Tour de France* History," a "comeback that defied logic." Inspired by Landis' epic ride, I finally purchased my first "road" bike (sort of—a sturdy tri-cross) that very afternoon (note: still not at work).

When Landis rode off on his Stage 17 breakaway ride, he embodied human "doing" at the edges of possibility. For American philosopher John Dewey, "doing" is the active response and organization of energies by humans "toward the world in a coordinated, discriminating way" (Alexander, 1998, 9). Active "doing" is intentional; it is human action seeking meaningful exploration of the lifeworld they exist within. Dewey uses descriptions such as "the going-out of energy," the act of "plunging into" a subject-matter (2008/1934, 59–60) to describe human "doing." Relatedly, Dewey's classic-pragmatism brethren, William James, similarly emphasized the centrality of human action to a meaningful existence. James wrote extensively on the strenuous life, whereby "'strenuous' connotes such vigorous active energy and robust effort, deriving from Latin and Greek words denoting activeness, vigor, keenness, eager desire, and exceeding strength longing to break forth into action" (Shusterman, 2012, 436). As contemporary American philosopher Richard Shusterman (2012) writes, "our human essence is more vitally active than rationally reflective" (434). We are, Shusterman continues, "more essentially active than rational creatures" (442)—thus human "doing" in endurance sports embodies a key feature of human existence.

Endurance athletes "doing" at the height of their powers evoke a kind of mesmerizing, motivational response from those fortunate enough to observe their feats. Historically great athletes in other sports, be it Michael Jordan in basketball, Serena Williams in tennis, Wayne Gretzky in hockey, Lionel Messi in soccer, or Nadia Comăneci in gymnastics, conjure up "did you see *that?*" performances, exerting their will on the "lifeworld" they function within, leaving us with a sense of awe at their physical exploits. But few can ever imagine performing at such levels in the highly technical and specialized crafts these generational sport figures operate within. Most of us, however, can connect with the relatively common physical acts of running, biking, or swimming. And while sprinting as fast as Usain Bolt for 100 meters, spinning around the severe embankment of a velodrome track like Laura Trott, or "butterflying" across the water similar to Michael Phelps is clearly unconscionable to most, elite endurance athletes like road cyclists, open water swimmers, and marathoners don't appear at first blush to travel using fundamental movement forms in "inhuman" ways. Subsequently, armadas of runners weave along urban paths on a daily basis and crowd the start lines of Sunday races, swimmers populate lanes wearing Speedos and stockpiling training devices on the pool deck, weekend warriors buy (tri-cross) bikes and stretch lycra to the limit to cycle country roads and climb hallowed hills. Endurance sport feats like Floyd Landis' Stage 17 ride, Paula Radcliffe's 2003 world record marathon run or Eliud Kipchoge's 2017 sub-2-hour marathon attempt, and volume contributor Scott Tinley's Ironman Hawaii victories in the 1980s reveal human possibility—*our* possibilities! And subsequently, they inspire us to run, to ride, to swim, to push our own limits, to see what *we* humans are capable of doing.[2]

But there is also an appreciation from enthusiasts that Landis on Stage 17, Radcliffe at the 2003 London marathon, Kipchoge on an Italian Formula I race track, and Tinley through Kona's Energy Lab—despite the supposed "simplicity" of their crafts—exhibited sustained physical exploits that "defy logic," seem "superhuman," and invoke the same "did you see *that*?" response normally reserved for feats in sports more suited to instantaneous brilliance. Anyone who has tried to maintain the pace of elite marathoners, professional bike riders, or competitive swimmers recognizes the gap between them and "the rest of us."[3] These high-performance endurance athletes use their bodies in effective and efficient ways reserved for only the best of the best. Athletes at the highest levels of sport perform inspirational feats of sporting prowess so magnificent the "weekend warrior" can only look on in awe and wonder. Perhaps more so than any other human endeavor, great athletes appear to "do" seemingly impossible, superhuman feats before our eyes. Great athletes use their bodies in time and space to publicly exhibit athletic acts seemingly perfect in execution, complete in efficiency, and startling in power. And they are able to push the bounds of possibility more than recreational athletes can imagine.

## THE AESTHETICS OF HUMAN "UNDERGOING" IN SPORT

But "doing" is only part of the story of sport and human performance (and human meaning) more widely. The reality is that no athlete, not Landis, Radcliffe, Kipchoge, Tinley, or Messi, Williams, Jordan, Gretzky, nor Comăneci, can function beyond the bounds of our lifeworlds. Great athletes, like the rest of us, are pushed to the ground by gravity, limited by the effects of heat and cold, wind and rain; the best athletes, not immune to human confines, must operate with restricted ranges of motion, constrained sense organs, and limited cardiovascular systems. Psychological demands will tax them, technical skills will fail them, tactics will disappoint them, rules will limit them, injuries will break them, age will "finish" them.

For instance, despite an apparent defiance of "regular" human limitations, even the world's greatest endurance athletes function at relatively low levels of "mechanical" performance efficiency. Laboratory tests on Lance Armstrong at the peak of his powers (1993–1999), for instance, measured his muscular efficiency levels—that is the amount of energy produced directed to the actual powering of his bicycle—consistently around 23 percent (Coyle, 2005; Gore, Ashenden, Sharpe, & Martin, 2008).[4] Similarly, elite 100-meter track sprinters, despite the relatively short distance travelled, must address their embodied limitations. As American sprint coach Harvey Glance observes, "It's not the person who accelerates the fastest who wins, it's the person who decelerates the least" (Arnold, Kelley, & Reynolds, 2008). Soccer-footballers over the course of a 90-minute match will push the limits of human performance due to maximum glycogen depletion and rising core body temperatures (Reilly, Drust, & Clarke, 2008). Even static target sports performed in relatively controlled environments—take darts for example—fall prey to the imprecision of human motor control and the psychological effects inherent to competitive situations.

But nothing exhibits the reality of human limitations more than elite endurance athletes, particularly those competing beyond the controlled confines of the bounded stadia. Like Landis on his disastrous final climb of Stage 16 at the 2006 *Tour de France*, elite Ironman competitors including Paula Newby Frazier, Julie Moss, Sian Welch, and Julie Ingraham[5] all famously hit the "wall" in Hawaii while challenging for the triathlon world championship, reduced to incoherent "human puddles" unable to even stand. These athletes tipped over the edge of their physiological capacities—that is the risk one takes in endurance sport. But human limitations in endurance sport extend beyond physical capacity into the mental, technical, and tactical realm. For instance, every Grand Tour is marred by crashes instigated through technical miscues by professional racers. Nairo Quintana, 2014 *Giro d'Italia* and 2016 *Vuelta a España* champion for instance, lost the lead of the Spanish Grand Tour in 2014 after crashing while fixing his shoe on a twisty descent.[6] Oscar Pereiro and other general classification contenders tactically misjudged Landis' breakaway, allowing him to ride away from them on Stage 17 and eventually win the *Tour de France*. Landis himself required a bike change in the midst of his epic breakaway while climbing the grueling Colombière due to a mechanical problem.

There is significant appeal to watching the greatest athletes confront human limitations such as thermoregulation, hydration, mineral depletion, forces such as gravity, biomechanical construction and degrees of freedom, fatigue, training capacities, as well as psychological unrest, tactical complexity, and technical complications. For instance, spectators at events such as the *Tour de France* typically seek out locales along the route where the suffering, the visible signs of human frailty, reaches an apex—normally on steep ascents near the course's finish line in the last days of an unrelenting stage race. Seeing an elite cyclist like Landis "bonk" on the final climb of Stage 16 is as much a part of the lure of endurance sport, its deep human meaningfulness, as his Stage 17 victory.

We want to see our sportspersons, especially top endurance athletes, pushed to the edge—to see them struggle, suffer, *endure*. When great athletes "tip over" this edge in the process of striving toward what Dewey refers to as an ever evolving "end-in-view," we often say they've been "humanized." Thus, the irrevocable complement to "doing" is, according to Dewey, "undergoing." "All experience involves some degree of 'undergoing' . . . the precarious aspect of existence is pervasive," writes Thomas Alexander (1998, 8). Even the greatest sporting champions must "undergo" in Dewey's language—they must be open to the world they find themselves constrained by, vulnerable to the limits of their being, finding outwardly directed needs unfulfilled (Alexander, 1998, 8). As Dewey asserts, "the first great consideration is that life goes on in an environment; not merely *in* it but because of it, through interaction with it" (2008/1934, 19).

Dewey considers human experiences of "undergoing," of limitation, of suffering in a broad sense, as essential for meaning and growth. Wong (2007), by way of Dewey, equates suffering (conceived of widely) with passion: suffering in this sense opens space to "experience intensely while being acted upon by the world" (202). To "undergo" involves a receptive appreciation of the obstacles, the limitations and inefficiencies, the inevitability of suffering thrown up by the lifeworld. "Undergoing" is thus to "let something happen to oneself and to bear the weight of its consequences" (Wong 2007, 202).

Dewey examined extensively the idea of humanity's sense of precariousness and its role in giving life depth. Our human frailties, the very real limitations we live with, give our endeavors meaning. Consequently, inefficiency and suffering provide portals through which humans may experience the world more aesthetically. In the end, human frailty, our destiny to feel the weight of helplessness, of limitation, of suffering on some level, is a gift. Our world, Lear (1999) argues, is fortunately a "good enough"—not a perfect or utopian—world and thusly provides a context in which deeply meaningful sport can exist. "In order to grow we must 'undergo,' that is, suffer. Life has depth because we can sense its precariousness," writes Alexander (1998, 8).

This is why activities ignoring the appeal of human limitations or suffering often fail to capture our attention long-term. Take as an example "Slamball"—a basketball-themed game played on a court with a series of trampolines designed to isolate athletes performing high flying maneuvers such as dunking the ball or blocking opponent's shots. Although Slamball athletes fly higher, perform increasingly spectacular dunks, engage in more powerful finishing moves than their basketball counterparts, the game ultimately lacks the appeal provided by the more bounded, inefficient original version requiring players to suffer against the weight of gravity in order to perform. Similarly, fans of the *Tour de France* are likely to find motorized versions of the race less interesting. Watching, for instance, motorcycles race over Pyrenees' mountain passes strips away human limitations and suffering, replacing them with less interesting, more sedate, mechanical challenges. So despite racing on the same course, on relatively similar machines, the replacement of inefficient human exertion with more efficient mechanical power bleaches the color (at least for endurance sport lovers) out of the activity.

Echoing Nietzsche, Dewey contends that the elimination (or denial) of the "goodness" of undergoing or suffering (in the broad sense) strips away "honest interactions" between humanity and the world (Wong, 2007, 215). "Our basic humanness," Wong (2007) concurs, "depends on suffering of this kind and is diminished in its absence." The vital necessity of "undergoing" for intensely meaningful experiences, Wong (2007) argues via Dewey, requires humans to relinquish conceptions of human meaning that assume our capacity to control the lifeworlds we exist within.[7] We cannot "will transformative experiences into being" (Wong, 2007, 204). So human meaning requires not only active "doing," but also receptive "undergoing"—we are "acted upon . . . often against our will" in intense uncontrolled ways (204).

In the end, suffering and inefficiency confirms that great endurance athletes *are* like us. Although we may cover less distance, move much slower, and only dream of accomplishing similar feats, Landis, and Radcliffe, and Tinley face the same human challenges (e.g., physiological and mechanical limitations), meet the same obstacles (e.g., difficult courses, inclement weather), suffer the same defeats (e.g., fail to meet expectations, endure injuries). The difference between them and us is in degree, not kind—and we value this embodied reality. Thus, to meaningfully live what James (1987) calls the "strenuous life," to fully realize our humanity, requires not only active doing but also strain, challenge, limitation—*receptive undergoing*.

## MEANINGFUL TENSION AND THE CENTRALITY OF AESTHETICS

Transformative moments in sport and beyond require an appreciation that an active tension or fusion between doing and receptive undergoing must exist (Shusterman, 2012, 436). Deep engagement does not happen when we merely act on the world or let the world act upon us. Doing and undergoing are "reciprocally, cumulatively, and continuously instrumental to each other" (Dewey, 2008/1934, 56). In an article connecting William James, endurance sport and suffering, pain, and loss, Anderson and Lally (2004) write "to engage in endurance practices—or any extensive physical training—is to choose a specific sort of physical suffering" (18). Undergoing has no existence disconnected from doing, it is not a dichotomous or dualistic relationship: "Undergoing is going out in order to receive; plunging in order to steep; pitching in order to take in" (Wong, 2007, 205). As Dewey writes:

> There are conditions to be met without which an experience cannot come to be. The outline of the common pattern is set by the fact that every experience is the result of interaction between a live creature and some aspect of the world in which he lives. A man does something; he lifts, let us say, a stone. In consequence he undergoes, suffers, something: the weight, strain, texture of the surface of the thing lifted. The properties thus undergone determine further doing. The stone is too heavy or too angular, not solid enough; or else the properties undergone show it is fit for the use for which it is intended. The process continues until a mutual adaptation of the self and the object emerges and that particular experience comes to a close. What is true of this simple instance is true, as to form, of every experience. (2008/1934, 43–44)

Importantly (and uniquely), this exploration of tensions, rather than search for clarity or certainty, stands as a key feature of the American philosophical project. In fact, Shusterman (2012) argues that the "strenuous mood" embodied in the aesthetics of tension, rather than the reflective rationality of traditional philosophy, defines pragmatism. Subsequently, pragmatists engage in inquiry for the purpose of exploring meaning rather than truth (in a final sense), accept they can only meliorate rather than solve problems, and seek out complexity rather than engage in a quest for certainty.

Peirce, in his work on evolution, picks up on this active tension between possibility and constraint, pointing to the necessity of malleable bounds for growth (Peirce, 1992; Elcombe, 2013). Evolution without form, he insists, is merely chaotic and random—and thus ultimately meaningless. Conversely, purely mechanical, predetermined conceptions of evolution fail to offer us a meaningful existence. If all of life were merely struggle, failure, and loss, then our lives would be empty. At the same time, if life mirrored the utopian vision constructed by philosopher Bernard Suits in his influential work *The Grasshopper*, whereby all of life's hardships fell by the wayside, then life would similarly lack depth and significance.

Instead, Peirce (1992; Elcombe, 2013) posits the notion of a developmental teleology, the fusion of order and capriciousness in his agapastic evolutionary theory. Merged with Dewey's ideas about doing and undergoing, pragmatists hypothesize that evolution occurs at the intersection of form and transformation. We, as humans in our practices such as sport, must appreciate and establish a vital harmony with the tensive world we are always already enmeshed within. All well-crafted sports, for instance, emphasize "optimal challenge" (Mandigo & Holt, 2002) creating a "sweet tension" (Fraleigh, 1984) between the possible and impossible. Ultimately, growth occurs at these edges of experience, at the messy tipping points where human doing and undergoing, efficiency and inefficiency, possibility and constraint meaningfully converge. A meaningful world requires simultaneous freedom and limitation—and what better context to appreciate this aesthetic ideal than within endurance sport?

For pragmatists such as Peirce, James, and Dewey, these kinds of "thick" aesthetic inquiries (Elcombe, 2017) serve a far more central role in philosophy than is often assigned. Typically reserved for narrow evaluations and conceptions of artistic creations, aesthetic discourse regularly sits on the philosophical sidelines in comparison with "real" inquiry into rational versions of ethics, logic, epistemology, and metaphysics. However, for Peirce, James, and Dewey, aesthetic tension lies at the heart of their American philosophical discourse. Aesthetics are primary for Peirce, James, and Dewey because, to them, it is about cultivating an experientially based awareness of our ideals. Much more than some determination of what is "beautiful," aesthetics *inquire into* that which embodied experience makes worthy of valuing. Art, Dewey argues, traditionally does the best job of this. Paintings, music, sculptures, poetry, more consistently than other forms of human action, immediately reveal meaningfulness in human experience in very social, and sometimes difficult, ways. But artfulness—or in Dewey's language, aesthetic experiences—is available in all human transactions with the world in which they are enmeshed. "The great moral to be learned from the arts for Dewey is that when ideals cease to be confined to a realm separated from our daily, practical experience, they can become powerful forces in teaching us to make the materials of our lives filled with meaning" (Alexander, 1998, 6). Cooking, teaching, gardening, building decks, engaging in conversations, riding bicycles, playing basketball, can all be performed artfully, creating opportunities for humans to experience "lift off the page" moments in even the seemingly ordinary or mundane moments of life (Elcombe & Tracey, 2010). Thus, Dewey's central challenge for humanity is to live more artfully, to engage in life filled with meaningful moments, to experience life aesthetically.

Importantly, the pragmatic view of aesthetics turns traditional philosophical inquiry on its head—aesthetics informing ethics, logic, and even metaphysics. For pragmatists, ethics pursues the "good" as it relates to our ideals. In other words, based on our experientially grounded ideals, what actions lead us to improve or make better what we do? Does Landis' use of banned substances enhance or detract from the meaningfulness of his ride? Similarly, logic pursues the melioration of our "truths" as they relate to ideals—with truth understood from a pragmatist perspective as "warranted assertions" rather than correspondence to some fixed reality. Therefore, if the aesthetic tension between doing and undergoing in directed human movement is a valued source of meaning and growth, an ideal that makes our life richer and deeper, then it should be used to inform what is "good" and what is "true" about sport.

## THE AESTHETICS OF TENSION AND THE IMPLICATIONS FOR SPORT

Consider how the aesthetic dimension of the tension between human doing and undergoing can affect sport ethics. Athletes at the highest levels cannot escape their embodied existence—they must "play" within the bounds of humanity. Technology, rules, training, tactics, can all reset the tipping point, adjusting what is considered possible and impossible. Most technologies in fact are designed in some way to play with our inefficiencies, to circumvent or limit them by resetting the doing/undergoing fusion. But when they seem to go too far, when the possible apparently overwhelms the impossible and doing engulfs undergoing, technologies are viewed as intrusive and disruptive of our sporting experience. Coming to working (not final!) agreements as to where to set and recalibrate the space where human inefficiency and efficiency should meet is a messy proposition. Does EPO use by endurance athletes, for instance, upset the "sweet tension" between the possible and impossible, or create new and preferred tipping points to explore? Engaging in an always ongoing normative process is thus necessary to adjudicate what actions are to be considered "good" in sport—what will get us more of what we want and less of what we do not want from athletic competition. As Dewey asserts, "growth itself is the only moral end" (2008/1920, 181).

Take, for instance, the central role fragility plays in providing meaningful depth to the fully human practice of sport. Interestingly, the nature of most sports requires athletes to subject themselves to a state of decline in order to optimize performance. A baseball pitcher, for instance, might throw mid-90s MPH fastballs, but at a greater risk of injury than if the same pitcher threw low-80s MPH fastballs. Similarly, the runner who pushes too fast in the first miles of a marathon or cyclist who attacks too early in a race cannot recover from the elevated levels of lactate generated in her system. But elite performance demands these athletes go to the edge of their possibilities, to risk going beyond their limits and breaking down—to give all and possibly end up with nothing. Since all athletes are "decelerating" in some ways during competition, the rate of deceleration (and the willingness to push the bounds of human limitations) is what generally differentiates success from failure.

But the centrality of limitation in sport extends well beyond performance events and into the training and preparation for elite competition. The tension generated by the Olympic Games' four-year waiting period, for instance, in large part influences its aesthetic appeal (its meaningfulness). Athletes have one chance every four years—dog years in an athlete's sporting lifespan—to "peak" in order to realize Olympic glory. Push too hard, go over the edge in training, sacrifice valuable time in the periodization schedule, and all is lost—athletes either race in less than optimal form, or in many instances fail to even qualify.[8] Consequently, endurance athletes need to build strategically, rest, recover, and taper with great care. Stay too far away from the edge, train too safely, however, and little will be gained when centimeters or seconds distinguish champions from the high performance "masses." This doesn't even take into consideration the pressure to perform at one's best during the competition. To endure four years of preparation for one single opportunity to perform almost perfectly provides much of the tension central to our aesthetic appreciation of sport. Consequently, the idea of accepting artificial, inefficient barriers in sport can go beyond the structure of games into the preparation for our competitions. Aesthetically, this seems to create growth, to make sport better, to give us more of what we want. Or maybe the fragility is too much, and technologies designed to enhance the athletes' resiliency (e.g., training recovery techniques) ought to be accepted to reset the doing/undergoing point of tension.

## THE CURIOUS CASE OF FLOYD LANDIS

Returning to Floyd Landis, the question we are left with is how should we view his Stage 17 performance? Should we still consider the ride, despite the eventual confirmation (and Landis' own acknowledgment) of the use of illegal means, one of the greatest in cycling history? On the one hand, Landis certainly performed an athletic feat lauded by experts and casual observers alike. With modern day tactics and training, despite Landis' poor placing at the start of the stage, strong general classification riders are rarely (if ever) allowed to escape from the main peloton. Landis, however, essentially rode a 120 km time trial without the assistance of other riders, effectively keeping increasingly nervous competitors at bay through to the finish. The expressions of his "doing"—determination, athletic courage, riding ability and apparent willingness to suffer at the limits of his being—continue to impress.

The appreciation for Landis' performance, based on what we know from science, must be tempered. In the moment and without knowledge of Landis' doping actions, he looks to be an athlete willing to suffer far more than his competitors, to push right to the precipice of human possibilities and limitations in pursuit of victory. Landis managed as an athlete, despite his inescapable frailty, to seemingly drive to the edges of human possibility, to undergo more than almost any other bicycle rider in a similar competitive context by accepting more pain, risking more physically and tactically, challenging the "norm" of how one ought to race.

But we cannot bracket out the impact the banned substances he took has on our aesthetic sense of that day's ride. Physiology and human performance research informs us that the kind of performance enhancement Landis' utilized likely helped him recover from physical distress from the disastrous Stage 16 in ways unrealizable without technological assistance. Consequently, evidence that he clearly suffered and risked more than the other riders becomes blurred. Those beyond the peloton can no longer assume that Floyd Landis went closer to the edge than everyone else, that what we watched was a human engaged in a human task at the limits of human possibility—at least at the limits we assumed existed without the experience of using certain performance enhancing substances. Lacking evidence to the contrary, all signs point to Landis extending the bounds of human frailty through the use of certain substances to a level currently deemed undesirable by those with a vested interest in the sport of cycling. In other words, Landis appears to have "moved the line" where doing and undergoing converge without "our" permission. The same aesthetic sense of tension lies behind decisions in sport to ban corked bats in baseball and square groove clubs in golf, to require bikes to meet a minimum weight for competition, and for swimmers' suits to meet certain buoyancy and permeability requirements.[9]

Yet, to add further complexity to the analysis of Landis, what if the others he competed against (as there are good reasons to suspect) were also "moving the [possible/impossible] line" by covertly doping? While the general public may not be privy to this manipulation of the tension between doing and undergoing, those within the peloton may not view Landis' use of banned performance as an unreasonable action. If we therefore compare Landis' Stage 17 ride to the "tipping point" between the possible and impossible accepted by the other professional riders that day (rather than our own amateurish conception where to draw the line), does our aesthetic sensibility, and therefore ethical assessment of Landis, change?

Within sport in general, and certainly endurance sport in particular, a clear central existential feature of competition is athletes pushing to some contingently defined tipping point of human possibility—with and without the aid of emerging technologies. Experiencing both the promise and limits of humanity, to see and feel "us" play at the edge of the possible and impossible, to do and undergo in extreme ways, provides deeply meaningful, fully aesthetic, "lift off the page" moments for both participants and spectators alike. And the process of arriving at working conclusions as to where we set those lines defining today's ideal of tension between human possibility and impossibility is not a "rational" task in the traditional philosophical sense—it is an aesthetic one.

This is why Floyd Landis serves as an ideal muse for the American philosophical project.[10] Rather than seek clarity, or certainty, or immutability, American philosophers working in the tradition of classical pragmatism break down clear dichotomies, search for meaning, explore tensions, find places for growth, and critique stagnation. Ultimately, we must recognize that our "warranted assertions" about the meaningful life (including those experienced through endurance sport) are aesthetic, rather than rational. Thus, aesthetic insights, including an appreciation of the tension between human doing and undergoing, should inform how we construct, adapt, transform, and assess our social practices. And true to the pragmatist project, no certainty is assured. Human activities will never be finished projects. But they can, if conceptualized aesthetically rather than rationally, contribute to deeper and more meaningful human existence.

## NOTES

1. The physical challenge required to compete in the Tour de France, one might argue, makes the use of performance enhancement techniques a necessity—including some banned forms—for the cyclists' health and well-being, subsequently shifting the responsibility from the athletes to the course organizers in terms of doping "coercion."

2. I argue children find such inspiration watching elite athletes in a wider range of sports. As we age we recognize the challenges more technically complex sports have and find inspiration in activities like endurance sports.

3. Although distance runners for instance, don't appear to be running fast, few people are capable of sustaining an elite like Ryan Hall's marathon pace on a treadmill: https://www.youtube.com/watch?v=ziQEsdXMbi8

4. Original study by Coyle (cited in Gore et al.) controversially suggested Armstrong improved muscular efficiency between 1993 and 1999. Coyle admitted calculation errors in his original study, and Gore et al. found further problems—and concluded his muscular efficiency remained consistent.

5. YouTube clips are available to see these high profile examples of "bonking," including Paula Newby-Frazier (https://www.youtube.com/watch?v=g_utqeQALVE), Julie Moss (https://www.youtube.com/watch?v=VbWsQMabczM), Sian Welch, and Wendy Julie Ingraham (https://www.youtube.com/watch?v=MTn1v5TGK_w)

6. YouTube video of Quintana's crash is available at: https://www.youtube.com/watch?v=aJr074MXqN8

7. The most influential example (from the psychological literature) is Deci and Ryan's self-determination theory. See E. L. Deci, & R. M. Ryan. (1985). *Intrinsic motivation and self-determination in human behavior*. New York: Plenum.

8. This in part explains the feeling of unease elicited when athletes claim "injury rehabilitation" as a defensible rationale for the covert use of banned substances.

9. See https://www.fina.org/sites/default/files/frsa.pdf for swimsuit regulations.

10. I am not suggesting Landis be viewed as a moral exemplar, but instead an ideal "lens" through which to explore the complexity of (pragmatically oriented) normative analysis.

# REFERENCES

Alexander, T. (1998). The art of life: Dewey's aesthetics. In L. A. Hickman (Ed.). *Reading Dewey: Interpretations for a postmodern generation* (pp. 1–22). Bloomington, IN: Indiana University.

Anderson, D. R., & Lally, R. (2004). Endurance sport. *Streams of William James* 6(2), 17–21.

Arnold, K., Kelley, A., & Reynolds, G. (2008, August 3). The Games, abridged. *Newyorktimes.com*. Accessed February 17, 2017: http://www.nytimes.com/2008/08/03/sports/playmagazine/803EVENTS-table-t.html

Coyle, E. F. (2005). Improved muscular efficiency displayed as Tour de France champion matures. *Journal of Applied Physiology* 98, 2191–2196.

Cycling News. (2006, July 20). Stage report/results. Cyclingnews.com. Accessed February 17, 2017. http://www.cyclingnews.com/races/tour-de-france-2006/stage-17/results/

Dewey, J. (2008/1934). *The later works of John Dewey, volume 10, 1925–1953: 1934, Art as experience*, J. Boydston (Ed.). Carbondale, IL: Southern University Press.

Dewey, J. (2008/1920). *The middle works of John Dewey, volume 12, 1899–1924: Essays, miscellany, and reconstruction in philosophy published during 1920*, J. Boydston (Ed.). Carbondale, IL: Southern University Press.

Elcombe, T. L. (2017). *Jogos Bonitos*? Sport, art, and aesthetics. In R. S. Kretchmar (Ed.). *Philosophy: Sport. Macmillan's interdisciplinary handbooks: Philosophy series* (pp. 299–317). Farmington Hills, MI: Macmillan Reference USA/Gale.

Elcombe, T. L. (2013). Agapastic coaching: Charles Peirce, coaching philosophy, and theories of evolution. In R. Lally, D. Anderson, & J. Kaag (Eds.). *Pragmatism and the philosophy of sport* (pp. 89–104). Lanham, MD: Lexington Books.

Elcombe, T. L., & Tracey, J. (2010). In J. Ilundáin-Agurruza, & M. W. Austin (Eds.). *Cycling—Philosophy for everyone: A philosophical tour de force* (pp. 241–252). Malden, MA: Wiley-Blackwell.

Fraleigh, W. (1984). *Right actions in sport: Ethics for contestants*. Champaign, IL: Human Kinetics.

Gore, C. J., Ashenden, M. J., Sharpe, K., & Martin, D. T. (2008). Data efficiency calculation in Tour de France champion is wrong. *Journal of Applied Physiology* 105(3), 1020.

James, W. (1987). The absolute and the strenuous life. In B. Kuklick (Ed.). *William James, writings, 1902–1910* (pp. 821–978). New York: Vintage.

Lai, G. (2006, July 20). Opinion: Landis topped LeMond, and Lance. *NBC Sports Online*. Accessed August 31, 2010. http://nbcsports.msnbc.com/id/13957633/

Lear, J. (1999). *Open minded: Working out the logic of the soul*. Boston, MA: Harvard University.

Mandigo, J. L., & Holt, N. L. (2002). Putting theory into practice: Enhancing motivation through OPTIMAL strategies. *Avante* 8(3), 21–29.

Murphy, A. (2016, July 7). Once among cycling's best Floyd Landis attempting to remake image. *SI.com*. Accessed February 17, 2017. http://www.si.com/more-sports/2016/07/07/floyd-landis-cycling-tour-de-france-doping

Murphy, A. (2006, July 3). Attitude on wheels. SI.com. Accessed February 17, 2017. http://www.si.com/vault/1969/12/31/8380964/floyd-landis-lance-armstrong-tour-de-france

Peirce, C. S. (1992). Evolutionary love. In N. Houser, & C. Kloesel (Eds.). *The essential Peirce: Selected philosophical writings, volume 1 (1867–1893)* (pp. 352–371). Bloomington, IN: Indiana University.

Reilly, T., Drust, B., & Clarke, N. (2008). Muscle fatigue during football match-play. *Sports Medicine* 38(5), 357–367.

Rego, P. (2009). *American ideal: Roosevelt's search for American individualism*. Lanham, MD: Lexington Books.

Shusterman, R. (2012). Thought in the strenuous mood: Pragmatism as a philosophy of feeling. *New Literary History* 43, 433–454.

Yarbrough, J. M. (1998). *American virtues: Thomas Jefferson on the character of a free people*. Lawrence, KS: University Press of Kansas.

Wong, D. (2007). Beyond control and rationality: Dewey, aesthetics, motivation, and educative experiences. *Teachers College Record* 109(1), 192–220.

*Chapter 4*

# Sunrise, Sunset

## *Reflections on What Makes an Aging Biker's Life Significant*

Scott Kretchmar

During my sunset years, the numbers have become less friendly. The rides are shorter. Times are slower. Recovery periods last days instead of hours. When I'm grinding up a hill on some off-road journey, there are moments when I'm not sure whose body I am occupying. Amputees have experiences of phantom limbs, but nobody told me about phantom bodies. Nevertheless, on this ride I seem to have found one. Old aspirations are still fresh. The world of hills, gravel roads, and considerable distances continues to issue familiar invitations. The body-self I once was reasserts itself. I push on with renewed hope and energy.

However, the wall appears before I am expecting it, that ubiquitous wall! Where did it come from? Why now? Why so soon? I think to myself this must be someone else's wall. How dare it threaten to ruin my ride?!

This experience and others like it have forced me to come to grips with reality. My bike is not the same friend she used to be. I've changed too. I cannot treat her as well as I once did, ride as many miles as we once rode, take her places I once took her. But it would be difficult to part ways. She and I have been together too long.[1]

My mountain bike is not just a metal object out in the garage; she has invaded my person. Because of her, my eyes see different things, my muscles present me with biking invitations, my aspirations and joys have been turned in biking directions. Many of my favorite stories include my friend. As a senior rider, and whether I wished it to be so or not, I have been thoroughly "biked." Moreover, I have returned the favor. My bike's well-worn tires, faded black paint, and scratches all bear testimony to my favorite rides, my goals, my skills, my personality. She has been thoroughly "Self'd" What an odd couple—an old biker and an old bike!

## JUSTIFICATIONS FOR BIKING COMMITMENTS

In some ways it is difficult to explain, let alone defend, relationships like these. Passionate, lifelong athletes have always had to find creative ways to justify their indulgences. Outsiders—those who have not been bitten by any sporting muse—suggest that it might have been better to devote what appears to be wasted play time and energy to more productive activities. While play is important, they might admit, it has to be kept in balance. And the lives of passionate riders are clearly unbalanced.

Outsiders might also point out the irrationality of seeking excellence in a physical domain that is more the province of youth, strong muscles, and uncompromised cardiovascular systems than aged bodies. They might say senior athletes are like inconsiderate guests at a dinner party. They lack the good graces and common sense to know when it is time to leave.

In short, aging bikers are left to reflect on the twin facts that they have given themselves to a seemingly insignificant activity and are now experiencing progressively lesser levels of success. Finding significance in senior-age biking would seem to be a tall order. Fortunately, William James attempted to answer this call. He did not write an essay on senior biking, but he attempted to penetrate the thick brush that obscures our view of worthwhile living.

James was not the first philosopher to ponder the nature of a significant life, but arguably he was one of the more sensitive scholars to do so. His essay on "What Makes a Life Significant" is tender, inclusive, and democratic in spirit. It would have us remove our culturally influenced blinders to gain a fresh vision of human nature and what counts as worldly success. He urges a "widening vision" in assessing human worth. "In God's eyes," he wrote, "the differences of social position, of intellect, of culture, of cleanliness, of dress, which different men exhibit, and all the other rarities and exceptions on which they so fantastically pin their pride, must be so small as practically quite to vanish" (McDermott, 1977, 650).

James contrasts such external assessments with his own preferred internal perspective. The superficial is associated more with the former, the humanly significant—the meaningful life—is tethered more tightly to the latter. To gain the perspective required for assessing significance, we need, in his terms, to "level down" the accoutrements of success and "level up" the importance of lived passions, virtues, and other subjective factors that, in turn, affect how we act toward the world.

# SPORT, EXCELLENCE, AND AGE: THE PROCESS OF LEVELING DOWN

Sport, from James' perspective, would be at high risk for distortions from external assessments. Sporting heroes are typically the fastest, strongest, most coordinated, and graceful athletes we observe. They have beautiful, well-proportioned, muscular bodies. They garner the most medals or championships. They make the most money. They seem to achieve the most fame and merit the most attention. And they are, for the most part, young! Sport is a domain for youth and the vitality that goes with it. World records are set by teenagers and 20- or 30-somethings, not 60-year-olds. Of course, someone who is 60 years old can set a record for . . . well, 60-year-olds, but this record always has an asterisk after it. It forever stands in the shadows of better performances, the best that our species can produce.

Perhaps this is the way it must be. After all, sport is a perfectionist pursuit. Sport is perfectionist in nature because it presents problems to be solved. Solutions that are better (closer to perfection) are inherently preferred to those that are worse (further from perfection). People are attracted to sport because they want to try their hand at addressing its various problems and addressing them well. Those who enter the fray with greater resources—better muscles, enhanced training, calmer nerves, greater flexibility—will start with advantages over those who have fewer virtues. In other words, they have greater perfectionist potential. In most sports, a well-trained 20-year-old will enjoy clear advantages over an equally well-trained 60-year-old.

This observation places a focus on a second feature of sport that favors the young. Sport is not only a perfectionist pursuit but also a conventional activity. That is, sports are constructed by us and for us. Sports are the product of their constitutive rules. Because we are the authors of the rules, we can test whatever cluster of virtues we wish to test. If we ever became bored or otherwise disenchanted with a game, we could change its rules . . . or simply trade it for a better game. When the card games Old Maid and "war" became tedious we traded them for bridge, *New York Times* crossword, or Sudoku puzzles. When tag became tedious, we turned to more complex games like football and soccer.

Here is where age comes back into the picture. We could construct sports that privilege 50- or 60-year-old bodies over those of 20-year-olds, but we do not do that. Or at least such games are typically not in the spotlight. In most cultures around the world, we privilege citius, altius, fortius, along with flexibility, faster reaction time, higher levels of $O_2$ uptake, and the like. In short, we build our athletic games to feature and celebrate young bodies and youthful capabilities.[2]

Because sports are constructed for young people, and often young males, adjustments need to be made when older citizens venture into these activities. In order to mask the fact that these modifications could well be interpreted as inferior forms of the genuine article, creative language is used to preserve self-respect. In golf, tees for 60-year-olds are not called "tees for the elderly" but rather "forward tees." High level competitions for golden agers are not called the "Old Folks Olympics," but rather "Senior Games." Nets are lowered, distances are shortened, fewer innings are played, equipment is modified. While the purpose of these modifications is defensible, the result is often demeaning. The Riddle of the Sphinx would seem to apply here. What rides on three wheels in the morning, two at noon, and four in the evening? Answer: The cyclist who moves from tricycle to bicycle and eventually to wheelchair.

James argued that the employment of external criteria leads to judgments that are narrow and only partially accurate, at best, and insensitive and insulting at worst. His analysis of what makes a life significant is a defense of the poor, blue collar workers, everyday mothers and fathers, those who never have been and never will be in the limelight. It is not a condemnation of the rich and powerful. They too can live lives of considerable significance, but it is the poor, the overlooked, who need a champion. They need a philosopher who can unravel the paradox of how an insignificant life can be genuinely significant. Aging bikers need a champion who can explain how a commitment to a seemingly insignificant practice that produces increasingly insignificant results can be significant.

Aging bikers are not the only physically active individuals who wait for such a defense. It would include those who are not physically gifted—many physical education students, recreational athletes, intramural players. It is also a defense of once-but-no-longer talented athletes in any sport—those who have been injured, have grown old, who enter local tournaments that nobody outside that neighborhood knows about but still cannot shake their habit and still play as if it mattered. As we will see, James' significant life is based on demanding criteria, but they cut across the boundaries of status, talent, power, notoriety . . . and age.

## LIFE *IN EXTREMIS*

James (1997) is a critic of mediocrity, comfort, security. He once visited Chautauqua, an educational center founded in 1874 and located on Chautauqua Lake in Southwestern New York state. He was impressed by the high culture he experienced there. He was so taken by its lovely accommodations and programs that his intended one-day visit turned into a week. He said

Chautauqua was a place of "sobriety and industry, intelligence and goodness, orderliness and ideality, prosperity and cheerfulness" (646). However, he also noted that this was a place that required "no effort." Near the end of his stay, he said he began thirsting for something "primordial and savage." He found the comforts of Chautauqua to be strangely unsatisfying. "This order is too tame," he concluded, "this culture too second rate, this goodness too uninspiring. This human drama without a villain or a pang: this community so refined that ice-cream soda-water is the utmost offering it can make to the brute animal in man" (647).

He identified precipitous living, strength and strenuousness, intensity and danger as the "strong flavors" of life. "Sweat and effort, human nature strained to its uttermost and on the rack, yet getting through alive, and then turning its back on its success to pursue another more rare and arduous still—this is the sort of thing the presence of which inspires us" (648). And surprising to himself, he found these very qualities in many common laborers, including peasant women. When he realized that such human "flavors" of living could be found in many walks of life, he reported that the "common life of common men began to fill my soul." Common folk, he said, are "our soldiers," "our sustainers."

## PLAYING WITH THE WALL: THE BIKER'S LIFE *IN EXTREMIS*

Every biker knows about the wall. In a sense it is our constant companion. We have to treat it with respect. It shows up in oxygen-depleted muscles, in our gasping for breath, in our aching shoulders. It tells us to shift down, take it slower, conserve our energy.

Playing with the wall is different from hitting it. The latter experience often signals the cessation of cycling—walking one's bike up a hill, calling for the sag wagon, sitting down to eat and drink. Playing with the wall is much more fun, and it takes several forms.

One game we play is called "Push Back." When we meet the wall on early rides, it seems to have a fairly deep and permanent foundation. However, during weeks and months of training we realize it is movable. We can ride faster and farther before the wall has its way with us. How far back can we push the wall? And how fast can we move it? Those are the questions, and those are the purposes of the game. When we push it further and more quickly than we ever believed possible, a delightful sense of closure overwhelms us.

A second game is called "Tease You." In this activity we attempt to ride perilously close to the wall without ever hitting it. We go out hard . . . but not too hard. We push ourselves to the limit . . . but not over the limit. We brush the wall from time to time and wonder if we can continue. But we do. We taunt the wall. We ride so close, we can smell its breath! We finish, and once again a deeply satisfying sense of closure overwhelms us. That is the closest to the wall, we tell ourselves, we have ever ridden.

Every biker has his or her own wall. The 20-year-old Olympian, the 45-year-old gravel rider, the 72-year-old road biker—all of them have personal walls. All of them can play "push back" and "tease you." All of them can experience the flush of excitement and accomplishment when these games go well.

This is the case because there is nothing absolute or fixed about walls. Likewise, there is nothing absolute or fixed about bikers. Whoever the biker is and wherever that biker's wall is, the challenge is there. The challenge awaits a response. Thus, all that is needed for living life *in extremis* is the desire, courage, and commitment to play with the wall.

## CONCERNS ABOUT DENIGRATING EXCELLENCE

James agreed that two sides characterize the significant life—our inner lives, on the one hand, and public actions and products, on the other. Visible, concrete success is important. No matter who the agent is, no matter what the project involves, effort must be rewarded with results, with progress.

This is true for young, competitive bikers, but it is true for older bikers, as well. When we ride, we are not satisfied simply with trying, with getting to some destination without some cardiac event. Our times do matter. The distances we can traverse also matter. When we compete, the places we finish in the race are important to us. But therein lies the rub. The actions and products of older bikers are inferior when compared with their own previous accomplishments and, even more so, when compared to elite standards of excellence.

Elite athletes might be compared to some of the visitors to Chautauqua—the polished, the intelligentsia, the well-to-do. To be sure, the best of these educated and powerful individuals accomplish things that impact the world for the better. Their position and power provide a foundation for producing outcomes that no peasant or common laborer could ever hope to produce.

In sport, gifted athletes are in much the same position. Only there is one difference. They have to be young. Paul Weiss (1969) is one of the most articulate spokespersons for this claim.[3] From his Platonic perspective, he waxed eloquent in his defense of excellence:

> Excellence excites and awes. It pleases and it challenges. We are often delighted by splendid specimens whether they be flowers, beasts, or men. A superb performance interests us even more because it reveals to us the magnitude of what

then can be done. Illustrating perfection, it gives us a measure for whatever else we do. (3)

Weiss is not adulating the relative excellence of an older athlete or even the prowess of young female athletes at the peak of their abilities. He makes this clear in his subsequent analysis. He suggests that "it makes good sense for a *young man* to want to be a fine athlete; it is not unreasonable for him to suppose that through his body he can attain a perfection otherwise not possible for him" (12, emphasis added). He asks rhetorically, why is sport so compelling? His answer: "Sport is attractive because it offers a superb occasion for enabling *young men* to be perfected" (19, emphasis added).

For James, external standards of achievement are not irrelevant. Meeting absolute levels of excellence—whether in athletics, business, politics or some other profession—does nothing to disqualify a person from having lived a significant life. In fact, James rails against the inequalities that existed in his time between the rich and the poor, a complaint that could be reiterated today. Excellence among well-meaning and talented politicians who affected social change would produce much good. But significance for James does not attach to excellence or momentous accomplishment. He put it this way: "If, after all I have said, any of you think they [significant social changes] will make any *genuine vital difference* on a large scale, to the lives of our descendants, you will have missed the significance of my entire lecture" (659, emphasis original). Significance has less to do with absolute accomplishment and more to do with effort, with living life *in extremis*. However, James goes on to make it clear, it depends on much more than that.

## THE MARRIAGE OF IDEALS AND VIRTUES

The significant life is not created by dogged determination alone. The hard labor of the defeated workman is not extolled by James (1977). Such a worker "feels no personal pride in [the work's] progress ... none of the joy of responsibility, none of the sense of achievement, only the monotony of grinding toil"(654). Similarly, the biker who sees his activity as a workout, who experiences biking as a duty, perhaps a fitness activity, may well miss the deeper significance of the sport. The laborer gets paid, and the older biker may get a bit healthier, but neither one will transcend the "monotony of grinding toil."

What elevates the expenditure of effort is something James called "ideal inner springs." Here is how he defined it:

> An ideal must be something intellectually conceived, something of which we are not unconscious, if we have it; and it must carry with it that sort of outlook,

uplift, and brightness that go with all intellectual facts. Secondly, there must be novelty in an ideal,—novelty at least for him whom the ideal grasps. Sodden routine is incompatible with ideality, although what is sodden routine for one person may be ideal novelty for another. This shows that there is nothing absolutely ideal: ideals are relative to the lives that entertain them. (656, emphasis original)

This is precisely the point that may be difficult to grasp in appreciating the significance of an aging biker's life. What may be "sodden routine" for the biker when younger is now "ideal novelty" for that same individual who has become a senior rider. In fact, older bikers are not without resources for producing fresh challenges. In other words, they have a number of ways to enliven their own ideal inner springs by reformulating their biking challenges.

One such reformulation might be called "The Endurance Challenge." Senior bikers are not inherently prevented from traversing great distances. It may take them more time to do so, but if they have sufficient courage, persistence, and resilience, such feats can be successfully undertaken. Cross-state rides are now common. Some vacation biking companies, both in North America and abroad, feature challenging rides for fit senior citizens. Organizations like the Adventure Cycling Association provide maps for rides that range from shorter in-state circuits to cross-country and cross-mountain-range rides. Adventurous senior bikers can now take advantage of bike routes on any continent and utilize the overnight hostels and other accommodations now available to support such rides. However the endurance challenge is formulated, and whatever form it takes, the goal is simply to persist and finish the ride.

A second reformulation of a biking challenge that can excite the "inner springs" might be called the "Distance Challenge." This is different from the endurance challenge because the biker has a limited amount of time during which to complete the ride. This follows the format of the so-called extreme competitions—those that establish seemingly impossible tasks that must be finished during fixed periods of time. During these events, if athletes lag behind, and it thus becomes apparent that they will not finish (or will not finish in the allotted time), they are pulled off the course. Often, participants will quit voluntarily.

Century rides are a common format for distance challenges. Riders begin in the morning and need to complete the 100 miles prior to nightfall or some other deadline. Another format that is appealing to senior riders is the gravel ride. An example is an event called the "Dirty Kanza." It is a 200-mile ride in one day, sometimes in the heat, sometimes in the mud, over mostly gravel roads in the Flint Hills of eastern Kansas. While this is technically a race, most senior riders have one goal—namely, to finish the ride within the allotted time. In a recent running of this race, 944 riders lined up for the event and only 553 finished the 200 miles prior to the 3 a.m. cutoff time.

A third formulation of ideals for senior riders is found in "The Self-Improvement Challenge." The most common structure for this involves repeating a distance while aiming to complete each successive ride in shorter periods of time. A variation is one of trying to maintain a high speed of travel or increasingly higher speeds of travel across varying distances.

Modern cycling technology assists in these challenges. GPS and other systems can provide extremely accurate measures of distance, rate of travel when moving, overall rate of travel (including stops), heart rates, energy expenditure, along with much other data. In short, resources for comparisons with previous rides are rich, accurate, and varied, and can serve to provide clear measures of personal improvement. The obvious goal in the improvement formulation is to better one's recent, previous performances.

These examples provide evidence for an important claim made by James, perhaps the closest he gets to sounding like an analytic philosopher.[4] Each of these formulations includes two elements—ideals and virtues. James (1977) argues that they are both necessary:

> The significance of a human life for communicable and publicly recognizable purposes is thus the offspring of two different parents, either of whom alone is barren. The ideals taken by themselves give no reality, the virtues by themselves, no novelty. (657)

The three exemplar challenges outlined above show that ideals are age-resistant. Senior bikers can always find ways to identify a meaningful goal or ideal. The only requirement is that it is a relevant challenge—not a perfect challenge, not a challenge that requires some absolute notion of excellence. It has to be a challenge that fits the cycling body that the senior biker currently lives toward these ventures. In spite of "phantom bodies" getting in the way once in a while, this process of adjustment is usually automatic and highly accurate. How we think, as Merleau-Ponty (1962) and others so clearly showed, is intimately connected to who we are. No objectification of the body, no external calculations are required. We do not first have to find our bodies and then deduce what they can do. New "just-right" problems present themselves automatically and are there for the taking.

Fortunately, the virtues are also age-resistant. James highlights the will to achieve as something that gives depth to the significant life. The will of a 2-year-old is known to be notoriously strong, but apart from that age anomaly, will is something that can be strong from our earliest days to our golden years. One could even argue that the will needs to be stronger for senior citizens who experience new pains and limitations. For instance, riding 100 miles with mild but painful hip arthritis requires a particularly robust will. Other requisite virtues of hope, persistence, patience, and the like can also be fully alive and well in senior athletes.

## IDEALS, VIRTUES, AND PROGRESS

One item is still missing from James' analysis, and he is unwavering on this point. It has to do with optimism, with expectations for progress or improvement. He criticizes Tolstoy's meliorism in adulating the pacific laborer, and he is equally dismissive of "orientalists and other pessimists."[5] James (1977) writes, "The thing of deepest—or at any rate, of comparatively deepest—significance in life does seem to be its character of *progress*, or that strange union of reality with ideal novelty which it continues from one moment to another to present" (657, emphasis original).

James calls this union that promises progress "strange," and elderly bikers can understand why. Progress for the senior biker can be unmistakably paradoxical. Successful rides, in other words, may seem to be decidedly unsuccessful from a logical point of view.

Performing repeatedly over weeks, months, and years at the same level—that is, not one second faster or one inch further—can be experienced as progress. (It would be normal, over time, for senior biking performance to decline.) Similarly, performing at lesser levels but with a slow rate of decline can also be experienced as progress. (It would be normal to see decline that is more rapid.)

Of course, progress can also include actual, objective improvements in performance. Physiologists have shown in multiple studies that elderly animals and humans can reverse certain effects of aging through diet, weight training, aerobic protocols, meditation, and other interventions. It is thus not uncommon to hear an avid senior biker report that he or she is performing better than was the case several years before. This may be a temporary victory, but it is a victory nonetheless. This is progress as we commonly understand it.

Senior biking is not a matter of putting up with the inevitable. It is not a matter of disconsolate waiting. Rather, it offers countless avenues for action, intervention, hope, dedication, and even progress.

## CONCLUSIONS

Previously, I described James' analysis of a life of significance as tender, inclusive, and democratic. These features of his work, I believe, come from the fact that he is a neutralizer. He neutralizes genetic/biological endowment. It matters little if one is tall or short, strong or weak, motor gifted or motor challenged, smart or unintelligent, young or old. He neutralizes social advantage: educated or uneducated, rich or poor, socially connected or left on one's own. He neutralizes position: powerful or weak; those with great responsibilities or those who do seemingly insignificant work. Perhaps most importantly, he neutralizes notoriety, the product of cultural judgment: those who are in lime light and those who are and will remain forever unknown. In a touching passage he talks about an encounter with some peasant women:

> Many years ago, when in Vienna, I had had a . . . feeling of awe and reverence in looking at peasant-women in from the countryside on their business at the market for the day. Old hags many of them were, dried and brown and wrinkled, kerchiefed and short-petticoated, with thick wool stockings on their bony shanks, stumping through the glittering thoroughfares, looking neither to the right nor the left, bent on duty. Envying nothing, humble-hearted, remote;— and yet at bottom, when you came to think of it, bearing the whole fabric of the splendors and corruptions of that city on their laborious backs. For where would any of it have been without their unremitting, unrewarded labor in the fields. (649)

James' essay does not feel like an academic treatise. It is more personal than that. He even urges his listeners and readers to "become more livingly aware of the depths of worth" that lie around them. He hopes his analysis will produce a little more humility and tolerance and reverence and love for others. The result, he argues, will be "a certain inner joyfulness at the increased importance of our common life" (658).

Old bikers should be beneficiaries of this humility and tolerance. Their rides too should be acknowledged as worthy accomplishments. To be sure, some seniors exhibit remarkable ability, uncommon skill levels, and garner victories in age-stratified cycling events. Some of them even finish well ahead of many younger competitors. But according to James, these offer no guarantees. He leaves the door open for another portrait of significance. It could be the dedicated senior biker, riding up some dusty mountain road, without accolades or notoriety and without much success as the world measures it, who has discovered what makes a life significant.

## NOTES

1. I am writing this essay from the perspective of a "serious biker." I fully realize that there are other more recreational ways to have "love affairs" with a bicycle. My analysis is not meant in any way to denigrate those other kinds of relationships.

2. This is analogous to the situation noted by feminist writer Jane English (1978) who argued that most popular games favor the male physique. Because games are

conventions, they could be otherwise. That is, games could be devised that are neutral to sex-typical physiques or even favor female athletes.

3. Michael Novak (1976) and Bob Simon (2015) are others who identify excellence as one of the central redeeming features of sport. However, Novak softens his stance by acknowledging the significance of virtues such as courage and persistence, and Simon is comfortable with relative notions of excellence that would accommodate fine play by elderly participants.

4. I find this curious because pragmatists are well-known for avoiding crisp, mathematical analyses. James stops short of saying these are necessary and sufficient conditions for the significant life, but this claim has that flavor. (See Kretchmar (2007) for a critique of analytic approaches in the sport philosophy literature.)

5. Some would argue that James' dismissal of eastern approaches to sport is too quick. To be sure, such perspectives as those provided by Zen Buddhism (see, e.g., Herrigel, 1964) would generate a very different portrayal of senior biking. Inherent in James approach are ego, desire, progress, and significance. All four of these factors would be sublimated in the calm, ecstatic Zen experience of "the bicycle riding itself." Perhaps more importantly, however, is the fact that the Jamesian approach is not necessarily at odds with Eastern traditions. Csikszentmihalyi (1990), for instance, argued that Zen-like flow experiences occur in a so-called flow zone, one in which challenges and skills are well-matched. James, in his own way, argues for the same—the matching of a person's capabilities with that person's projects. Thus James, on my reading, would actually expect life *in extremis* to include, at least occasionally, flow experiences.

## REFERENCES

Csikszentmihalyi, M. (1990). *Flow: The psychology of optimal experience.* New York: Harper & Row.

English, J. (Spring, 1978). Sex equality in sports. *Philosophy & Public Affairs* 7(3), 269–277.

Herrigel, E. (1964). *Zen in the art of archery.* New York: Pantheon Books.

James, W. (1977). What makes a life significant. In McDermott, J. (Ed.) *William James: A comprehensive edition.* Chicago, IL and London: The University of Chicago Press, pp. 645–660.

Kretchmar, S. (2007). Dualisms, dichotomies, and dead ends: Limitations of analytic thinking about sport. *Sport, Ethics and Philosophy, 1*(3), 266–280.

Merleau-Ponty, M. (1962). *Phenomenology of perception.* Translated by Colin Smith. London: Routledge & Kegan Paul, New York: The Humanities Press.

Novak, M. (1976). *The joy of sports: End zones, bases, baskets, balls, and the consecration of the American spirit.* New York: Basic Books.

Simon, R., Torres, C., & Hager, P. (2015). *Fair play: The ethics of sport.* 4th ed. Boulder, CO: Westview Press.

Weiss, P. (1969). *Sport: A philosophic inquiry.* Carbondale, IL: Southern Illinois University Press.

## Chapter 5

# Representative Endurance Athlete

Peter Hopsicker

In many ways, Ralph Waldo Emerson's collection of essays, *Representative Men*, examined the notion of genius—the idea that there are persons of exceptional intellectual or creative ability who in their characteristics and actions answer questions that ordinary people do not even have the skill to ask (Emerson, 1996, 5; Gura, 1977, 382). First published in 1850, Emerson provided six examples of "great men" who demonstrated their unique capacity to refine the raw essences of nature into ideas, and then into actualities, transforming them into new and vitalized improvements of the world. Each of these "representatives" answered questions "which none of his contemporaries put" (Emerson, 1996, 5), revealing a certain aspect of nature to others who had not the capacity to do so, resulting in some sort of amelioration of humankind.

Emerson's defense of the representative genius, specifically of Plato, Swedenborg, Montaigne, Shakespeare, Napoleon, and Goethe,[1] could be considered outdated. His ideas on genius should certainly be consumed within his historical context. As fate would have it, Emerson did not live during the same era as Albert Einstein, the iconic exemplar of genius in modern times. Even so, the idea that certain individuals possess abilities to ameliorate specific aspects of the world remains central to the ongoing pursuit of identifying and understanding genius (McMahon, 2013; Kalb, 2017).

Definitions of genius remain elusive and subjective. It is not my goal to suggest one here. This definitional obscurity, however, allowed for the discussion of genius to expand into human sporting practices. Often couched alongside examinations of athletic excellence as a function of genetic predisposition (see Epstein, 2013; Brenkus, 2010), cultural advantage (see Coyle, 2009; Colvin, 2008; Gladwell, 2008), or creative behavior (see Hopsicker, 2011; Lacerda and Mumford, 2010), literature in recent decades demonstrates a growing interest in considering exceptional human motor behavior as genius.

Examples of sporting genius tend toward the exceptional performance of complex motor behaviors. Dustin Johnson (golf), LeBron James (basketball), Sidney Crosby (hockey), Lionel Messi (soccer), and Venus or Serena Williams (tennis) are often cited. From an Emersonian perspective, one could argue that these individuals are "representative" of their sporting practices. They solve sport-specific problems in novel and creative ways, refine the raw nature of human movement into something more special, more exciting, and more revealing of the world, and ultimately exemplify genius through their demonstrated athletic talents. Endurance sports athletes rarely grace this list. Why?

Perhaps it is because endurance athletes (I refer specifically to runners and cyclists) occupy a sort of paradoxical place in the sports world. On the one hand, the endurance athlete's basic activities are very commonplace. We all learned to run and experienced running early in life. It is a readily accessible basic motor skill. The same could be said for cycling. While not everyone owns or has ridden a bicycle, the machine's ubiquity throughout the world provides ample evidence to consider bike riding, like running, as a familiar and shared human experience. This acquaintance and sharedness cannot be said for more specific sport skills such as the basketball jump shot, the soccer instep drive, or the golf swing. Perhaps it is the familiarity with endurance activities and the subsequent perceived simplicity of its core skills, the repetitive performance of the same motor action over and over again, that precludes such activities from genius consideration.

On the other hand, running and cycling can be considered very foreign and complex experiences. Empathy with these basic motor behaviors quickly erodes when they become purposeful activities measured in distance and time. In contrast to our uncomplicated comprehension and ability to run, most do not have experience with running over extended distances and time nor do they phenomenologically understand the running of a half-marathon, marathon, or ultra. Similarly, while "it's just like riding a bike" to most, few have taken bike rides beyond the comfort of their neighborhoods, performed century rides, or participated in *gran fondos*. Only the exceptional have experienced multistage events such as the Tour de France. Ironically, while we almost universally understand what it is to run and bike, most cannot comprehend those same activities when pursued as "endurance activities"—that is, when pursued with the goals of covering specific distances evaluated by measured amounts of time.[2]

Yet do demonstrated endurance efforts of bipedal ambulation (running) or human-powered vehicle operation (cycling) directed at covering significant distances in the shortest amount of time really "answer questions that ordinary people do not even have the skill to ask"? According to Brenkus (2010), sport science has already answered, or at least predicted the answer to, the endurance running question. He posits that a human graced with the "perfect" physiology will someday run a sub-two hour marathon (207–222). Organizations, such as the SUB2HR Marathon project (www.sub2hrs.com; Caesar, 2015), vigorously pursue that goal. Provided the ever-growing body of sport science literature, one could also assume that the predicted maximum for cycling's hour record, the longest distance cycled in one hour (www.cyclingweekly.com/tag/hour-record), could also be resolved. While this may be an oversimplification, and I am certainly not suggesting that the achievement of these limits is not in line with the internal goods of the endurance sports practice, the asymptotic nature of human motor performance strongly suggests predetermined "answers" to many endurance sport questions—questions delimited by the human physiological factors of height, weight, arm and leg length, and $VO_2$ max, to name a few.[3] Given the limits of the flesh and the growing predictive properties of sport science, can we say that those who strive and approach achievement of these "known" limits deserve consideration on the list of sporting geniuses? Should they be the "representatives" of endurance sport?

In the following pages, I seek to explore the idea of Emerson's "representativeness" in endurance sport. What do representatives of the endurance sport practice reveal in nature and how do they ameliorate the world through their actions? During this exploration, I will both side with Emerson and depart from him. First, while the representative qualities of endurance sport may require attention to distance and time, I will argue that they alone do not provide a sufficient description of the "nature" of the practice nor a sufficient account of what is revealed to others through its endeavor. Second, I will depart from Emerson and sidestep the identification of a specific "representative endurance athlete." Rather than identifying a representative person, I will suggest a representative endurance community. Conclusions will suggest that the representativeness of endurance sport—the genius—does not reside in the performance measurements of time and distance, but rather in the ameliorating relationship between the mover and the non-mover.

## EMERSON'S ANGLE OF VISION

In his essay "The Natural History of Intellect," Emerson described life as an "angle of vision." "A man is measured by the angle at which he looks at objects," he wrote. "What is life but what a man is thinking all day? This is his fate and his employer. Knowing is the measure of the man. By how much we know, so much we are" (www.rwe.org/the-natural-history-of-inte

llect). Essentially, Emerson believed that a person's viewpoints and actions are shaped by their experiences—shaped by what they know and how they employ that knowledge to the world.

Emerson shared an "angle of vision" with the transcendentalists of the nineteenth century. He believed that humans and nature complemented each other. Humans refined the raw essences of nature into ideas, and then into actualities, transforming them into new and vitalized improvements of the world. Each individual had certain capabilities to reveal a part of the world, and each human would, ideally, spend his or her life searching, finding, and using his or her own unique purpose.

"Representative" persons exemplified those who were exceptionally talented at revealing and ameliorating specific aspects of the human experience—by illuminating a certain aspect of nature to others. However, Emerson expected more than revelation from these individuals. He did not believe that "great" persons simply imparted a way of life to be followed. Rather, he believed in a dialectical relationship that not only revealed nature in all its glorious truth but also empowered others with the insight to reorient their lives for the betterment of the world. Great persons, he wrote, "cleared our eyes from egotism, and enabled us to see other people and their works" (Emerson, 1996, 15). Emerson sought not only that which these "representatives" brought to the equation but also the transformation of their ideas into changes beneficial to the self and to the world. Emerson worked within this transformation.

Emerson also valued effects over sources with a "nervous discontent with all received wisdom" (Emerson, 1996, x). He encouraged active participation in the exchange of knowledge between "representatives" and others and implored us not to simply be "sacks and stomachs" of wisdom (Emerson, 1996, 8). The value of representative persons, he suggested, emanates from the effect they have on how others live their lives to further achieve and reveal the greatness of nature in their own unique way. Subsequently, the amelioration and reorientation of the representative's ideas are directed toward that which others are destined to reveal. This dialectical relationship that Emerson proposed minimized distinctions between giver and receiver while it maximized the importance of transmission or communication of ideas and thoughts from one person to the next.

## THE ENDURANCE SPORT ANGLE OF VISION

Endurance athletes also share a common "angle of vision" as they reveal specific aspects of nature to the world. Qualities such as cardiovascular measures, nutritional requirements, training schedules, and a shared attention to time and distance (to name a few) can be found within both the running and cycling communities. Within this broad stroke of endurance sport knowledge, however, there appears to be three noteworthy "angles of vision": joggers/riders, runners/cyclists, and athletes[4] (Smith, 1998).

Joggers and riders, those most likely possessing the least commitment or competitive fervor for the practice, "train infrequently, race episodically (if at all), and only did either if the weather was fair" (Smith, 1998, 176). The straightforward goals of "body maintenance"—weight loss, fitness, and "looking good"—are the common motivations for this group (Smith, 1998, 176). Athletes, whether on foot or on bike, live a significantly contrasting perspective. They are the elite, potential winners of competitive races. Guided by distinctions of winning and losing, high rankings, and reputation among small groups of elite performers, athletes exemplify the discipline and dedication required to traverse distances in the shortest amount of time (Smith, 1998, 175–176).

In between the joggers/riders and the athletes is the faction of runners and cyclists who "train week in and week out at levels far in excess of that required for basic physical fitness, yet stand no realistic chance of winning or doing well in *any* race" (italics original; Smith, 1998, 176). Like Emerson's "Skeptic" Montaigne, runners and cyclists "occupy the middle ground," "finds both (athletes and joggers/riders) wrong by being in extremes," and "labour to plant their feet, to be the beam of the balance" (Emerson, 1996, 88). Committed to the practice more than the jogger/rider but not to the performance extremes of the athlete, these are the "also-rans" whose usually vague reasons for participation revolve around a "personally defined measure of satisfaction" such as personal records (PRs) or rank within age-classifications (Lockhart, 2010).[5]

These "angles of vision" reveal the nuances of purpose within the endurance sport community. From those purposes we can begin to discover potential endurance sport "representatives." With little doubt, athletes may be the *prima facie* candidates. Smart money certainly backs the athlete achieving the predicted limits of human endurance performance, but is this truly "representative" of this practice? As myself and the editor of this volume have argued elsewhere, achievement of those specific internal goods of the endurance sport community requires what American philosopher William James calls an "unsympathetic attitude" toward anything but attaining those goals (Hopsicker and Hochstetler, 2014). The athlete's angle of vision and subsequent behavior sways little from this focus. As noted above, however, the limits of human flesh and the predictability of those outcomes diminish the "revealing" and ameliorating nature of that pursuit. Are athletes transforming the "raw essences" of nature into ideas and then into improvements to the world or are they simply striving to demonstrate a known outcome?

Of course, joggers and riders are in no position to physically approach the human endurance limits defined by distance and time.[6] With all due respect to those of this angle of vision, I believe Emerson would accuse them of being "sacks and stomachs" (Emerson, 1996, 8) of endurance sport knowledge, of accepting that which was achieved by runners, cyclists, and athletes as if through "the pores of the skin" (Emerson, 1996, 15), and of failing to understand that the "best discovery the discoverer makes for himself" (Emerson, 1996, 16). Simply, joggers' and riders' dabbling with endurance activities rarely reveals anything new in nature nor exemplify a reorientation toward the amelioration of the world to any representative degree.[7] While Emerson understood that the reception of knowledge in any practice often happened in an unlimited, thoughtless, and relatively easy manner, he found fault with those who did not seek to utilize that knowledge in productive ways. Joggers and riders, after accepting the revealed knowledge from the other angles of vision, seemed to "stop where they stop. Very hardly can (they) take another step" (Emerson, 1996, 15) and use that knowledge to further ameliorate the world.

Ironically, runners and cyclists strive in endurance activities to a significantly more intense degree than joggers and riders. Yet these individuals participate with the complete knowledge of that which they cannot attain—demonstrating the limits of human endurance potential or even winning any particular race. Ultimately, runners and cyclists may be more interested in the process of sport rather than any particular competitive outcome (see Hochstetler, 2003). Still, while runners and cyclists exhibit a passion for endurance activity that will rarely if ever afford them "greatest of all time" accolades,[8] participation in running activities (including trail running) remained the most popular outdoor activity among Americans in 2016 (51.5 million participants) while bicycling activities (road, mountain, BMX) were the second favorite (43.1 million participants) during that same year (Outdoor Foundation, 2016, 11).

While these reports give no indication of the intensity of the running and cycling activities, it does appear that a large segment of the population seeks ongoing experience with endurance activities beyond the dabbling of the jogger and rider but not at the focused intensity of the athlete. In fact, between 2013 and 2016, competitive U.S. running events have experienced a drop in "finishers"—from more than 19 million in 2013 to fewer than 17 million in 2016 (Bush, 2017). Fewer people are toeing the starting line. Perhaps this demonstrates that competitive racing and the potential of winning are unsustainable motivations for most runners and, almost certainly, most cyclists.

## THE REPRESENTATIVE RUNNER AND CYCLIST

Given this overview, if we look for representativeness in the broader endurance sports practice, within which cadre of performers would that representation reside? Joggers and riders do not appear to have a significant embrace of the practice to be considered. While they may understand endurance sports questions, they are either unmotivated or are simply in a different stage of their lives to answer them to any ameliorating degree. Athletes, while highly engaged in the project of conquering the challenges inherent in human-powered locomotion, sport science may have already answered the questions for them. The answers to how fast a human can run or cycle a particular distance appears to be predictable and known. All that is required is a physiologically "perfect" human specimen. Would we not expect the representative of endurance sport to represent more than calculations of human-powered distance and speed?[9]

Of course, this leaves runners and cyclists—those who are deeply engaged in the endurance sport experience yet lack the specific qualities or opportunities that would characterize them as elite. Why should we look within this angle of vision? I would suggest that the answer alludes to a quality that Emerson noted about Shakespeare, his "representative" of the "power of expression, or of transferring the inmost truth of things into music and verse" (Emerson, 1996, 122). Emerson noted that Shakespeare:

> knew that a tree had another use than for apples, and corn another use than for meal, and the ball of the earth than for tillage and roads; that these things bore a second and finer harvest to the mind, being emblems of its thoughts, and conveying in all their natural history a certain mute commentary on human life. (Emerson, 1996, 124)

I suggest that endurance sports have a "use" other than the "body maintenance" goals pursued by the jogger and rider or the attainment of a human "perfection point" by the athlete—a formula determined by distance and time limited by physiology.

I suggest that runners and cyclists are representative of the endurance sport practice. In contrast to the jogger/rider and athlete, I believe runners and cyclists are not primarily in the business of conquering or overcoming time and distance and instead create and embrace both. Of course, the metrics of time and distance are important and applicable to all three angles of vision—even if only as part of the most basic description of one's performance, for example, "I ran for 30 minutes this morning" or "I rode 30 miles today." Yet the runner and cyclist "use" the miles and minutes of endurance activities to reveal aspects of nature in ameliorative ways in contrast to the jogger/rider and the athlete who consider those minutes and miles as things to be overcome in very specific and constrained ways.

For example, in his chapter titled "The Phenomenology of Becoming a Runner," J. Jeremy Wisnewski (2007) described a self-imposed movement experiment. As a nonparticipant in endurance sport, Wisnewski endeavored to "become a runner" and through that process determine if becoming a runner would ultimately alter his experience of the world. He concluded that it did, but not in the ways he expected. While this novice jogger admitted to initially experiencing a transformed perception of the world, a world he now perceived in terms of minutes and distance, Wisnewski described those minutes and miles as "decidedly unpleasant." To him, jogging constituted a "phenomenology of obstacles." Time and distance were simply things that "stood in the way" of his "rest" and "bodily peace" (37–38). For this jogger, time and distance were at the core of the "inertia of a non-runner" (37). They were obstacles to be pushed through, and he feigned no interest in creating more of it or embracing the experience.

Competitive athletes also perceive time and distance as obstacles to be overcome but not in the same way as subduing the "inertia of a non-runner." From the athlete's perspective, time and distance constitute the core variables of a mathematical formula in need of resolution. They are the variables that athletes impatiently seek to vanquish. Like explorations into outer space or to the deepest parts of the ocean, humans have waged an ongoing effort to conquer specific truths of nature to constantly redefine our place in the world. Human-powered locomotion is one of them. At the extreme of this quest is the SUB2HR Marathon project whose objective is to have a man run a full marathon in less than two hours within the next five years through the deciphering of a formula—"a dedicated scientific approach involving the very latest knowledge in key areas such as genetics, bioenergetics, biomechanics, nutrition, sports engineering and coaching and performance science" (www.sub2hrs.com/the-science/). As indicated above, sports science has in many ways determined the solution to that formula. All that is needed is a physiologically perfect human trained in scientifically based endurance practices.

Yet even short of this extreme, the athlete mentality always appears to be directed at defeating distance and time—a mentality that ultimately seeks, no matter how outlandish the idea, the completion of any long distance with a finishing time of 0:00. The existence of the "personal record" or PR in endurance athlete parlance attests to these efforts to overcome these consummate realities. Disgraced American cyclist Lance Armstrong (2001) provided such a perspective:

> I'd never ridden just to ride . . . there had to be a purpose behind it, a race or training regimen. . . . I wouldn't even consider riding for just thirty minutes or an hour. Real cyclists don't even take the bike out of the garage if it's only going to be for an hour-long ride. (144)

Olympic athlete Ted Corbitt echoes Armstrong's perspective when he notes how finishing his first marathon immediately got him thinking about how he could improve his time on the next one (Corbitt, 1998, 83).

Utilizing Emerson's assessment of Shakespeare, it seems that the jogger/rider and the athlete do not see endurance activities for any other "use" than overcoming distance in the shortest amount of time through human-powered locomotion. Their scientific materialism perspectives lead to very simple understandings of the endurance sports practice via data-driven cause and effect deductions.[10] The jogger/rider may desire the results of her "body maintenance project" through the participation in endurance activities, but ultimately wants the activity to be over so she can move on to whatever is next. Athletes also want to complete the activity in the shortest amount of time but do so with asymptotic goals and ongoing recalculation aimed at faster PRs in future efforts.

To be sure, runners and cyclists are certainly attuned to the experiences of time and distance. Like the athlete, they may at times pay particular attention to completing specific foot races in the shortest amount of time and act according to those goals. At other times, like the jogger/rider, they may simply just want to complete the day's mileage and move on to the next thing.

Yet I would suggest that runners and cyclists find meaning in endurance sport's centrality of distance and time that is often distinct from the jogger/rider and the athlete. Like Wisnewski, their perspectives on the world grow to include distance and time as principal organizers of life, but in a significantly different way. They do not seek to find ways to conquer the miles; they seek ways to accentuate and cultivate them and pass those experiences on to others.

The cyclist from the perspective of riding in a car, for example, consciously reviews the qualities of the road, the depth of the road's shoulder, the steepness of the grade, and the flow and amount of traffic (among other things) not necessarily to determine how the stretch of road would contribute to achieving faster times. Rather, the cyclist reviews such qualities to assess if this would be "a good place to ride"—one that would provide a high quality physically sensuous experience (Hopsicker, 2010). In a similar way, the runner travelling away from home seeks running routes that go beyond the need to complete the miles in a specific training program. Instead, the miles serve as a way to explore new places, see the cultural landscape firsthand, and provide opportunity for spontaneous and sometimes precipitous encounters.

Two personal examples may help clarify my point. I consider myself a runner. During a recent vacation to Ocean City, Maryland, I ran to the state of Delaware—a mere mile and a half from my hotel via the beach. I started my run before sunrise, completed the distance to the Maryland-Delaware boarder, and then continued to run north over the beaches of Fenwick Island. I kept running until only I made footprints in the sand. Then I ran a little farther and was alone. I created the run as I ran it. I had no idea the distance I ran and my pace was irrelevant. I had no preconceived plan to overcome the challenges of running in the sand nor did I have any desire to leave those challenges behind me. I reveled in experiencing the breaking of a new day, the glimpses of dolphins just off shore, and an encounter with a seal taking a break on the sand on his way to points further south—experiences missed by less movement-oriented friends. I ran the run not primarily as a means to some other goal, but as an end in itself. I "used" the run as a way to demonstrate that the beach was for something more than denoting earth from water. I "used" the run to reveal qualities of experience often overlooked as mundane and ordinary by others.[11]

I also consider myself a cyclist both on the road and on the trails. Near my home are the Allegrippis Trails[12] which I regularly mountain bike each Friday during the summer. I make every effort to be at the trailhead by sunrise. This essentially allows me to be the first on the trails for the day and to be alone for most of my ride. Both are more important to me than the mileage I ride and how fast I ride it. Being the first in the woods means an increased likelihood that I will encounter wildlife—primarily white-tailed deer and gray squirrels, but also the occasional box turtle or black bear. I can always tell that I am the first on the trails by the number of spider webs that I encounter during my journey. Created during the night between the trees growing on either side of the trail, I often unwillingly break them with my face, a sensation that isn't for everybody. Yet it is sensations and experiences like this that are my own creations of distance and time, not my attempt to overcome them. To be sure, I do describe my rides to my friends in terms of distance and time, but I spend significantly more time describing the cool mist of the morning, the dizzying shadows created by the sun rising through the trees, and the ephemeral yet profound sensations of solitude I experience within those constraints. I am not intolerant with the miles or my time on the trails. In essence, I create and embrace the attributes of that distance and time. My goal is not to conquer and leave those miles behind. My goal is to "use" those miles as my own creation and to bring my encounters to life with others unfamiliar with such experiences.

I am certainly not suggesting that I am the representative endurance athlete! In fact, counter to Emerson, I do not believe that any one person can do so. Instead, I suggest the existence of a representative endurance sports community, a goal more aligned with Philip F. Gura's (1977) work, "Thoreau's Maine Woods Indians: More Representative Men." Gura criticized Emerson for "failing to abide by his own egalitarian proposition" (366). Rather than adhering to his declaration that representative persons "must be related to us" (Emerson, 1996, 5), Emerson instead fixated on six "great men"—the "intellectual giants" of Plato, Swedenborg, Montaigne, Shakespeare, Napoleon, and Goethe (Gura, 1977, 366), men far removed from the activities of the masses.[13]

Gura suggests a more corporate yet democratic understanding of Emerson's claims. He examined Henry David Thoreau's biographic sketches of the nineteenth-century Penobscot Indian guides of the Maine woods, and contended that Thoreau, once a disciple of Emerson, was just as interested in "discovering and defining representative men for his age" (376). Through his examination of Thoreau's writings, Gura suggested that Thoreau believed the Penobscot Indians represented a community who could "read the poetry and mythology of his environment" and who knew "in the deepest sense the *anima* of the land he inhabited" (italics original, 381). While Thoreau employed Joe Polis (a Maine guide and Penobscot Indian) as the central figure in his biography, unlike Emerson's great men Polis was understandably more related to "us" having "founded no religions, written no great books, (and) conquering no continents" (381). Furthermore, Thoreau appeared to generalize the "representative" nature demonstrated by Polis to all Native Americans, broadly characterizing them as representative of "a vigorously healthy and cosmically symbiotic relationship with nature"—one he felt was critical to "a nation rapidly forgetting its relation to the land which defined its uniqueness" (368).

The running and cycling community's "angle of vision" provides the most fertile ground for the existence of an endurance sport "representative." It is an "angle of vision" that transcends the basic premise of endurance sport—the traversing of long distances in the shortest amount of time. Together, they represent the idea that movement is important beyond the times and miles completed. They represent a "use" for movement beyond practical and utilitarian applications. As such, they would agree with Emerson's assessment of "our impatience of miles, when we are in a hurry" when he adds, "but it is still best a mile should have seventeen hundred and sixty yards" (Emerson, 1996, 44). Runners and cyclists "use" the time and distance as a way to reveal to others the qualities of those minutes and miles that have evolved overtime into either monotonous and easily dismissed activity (from a jogger/rider perspective) or mundane measurements directed at fixed outcomes (from an athlete perspective).

Runners and cyclists ameliorate the world by demonstrating that even a commonplace activity that does not seek external reward can still reveal qualities of life that keep us tethered to our humanity. Anderson (2001) advocates a similar conclusion when he suggests that movement and sport can help us recover our "inner wildness" important to maintaining our humanity. He also notes that "the tamest-looking sports" (142), including walking, are sites for such "inner wildness" to occur. As such, running and cycling, while ordinary and shared experiences, cannot be easily dismissed as irrelevant or unnecessary even when performed for their own sake.

Anderson's conclusions, however, need to be retooled to an Emersonian perspective. While experiencing and revealing our own "inner wildness" to ourselves is an amelioration of its own kind, Emerson expected us to pass that which is revealed on to others so that they may be empowered to reorient their own lives for the betterment of the world. I would suggest that this dialectical relationship between the runner/cyclist and others is often hindered by unnecessary and unrealistic expectations.

For example, when the athlete advises the jogger to sign up for the "bucket-list" marathon, I wonder if progress is stunted. In some cases, this suggestion is veiled with hints of pretentiousness. To the point is Atkinson's (2008) examination of the triathlon culture. Within his findings, he notes how "the thin and fit triathlon body has become a symbolic representation, especially during a time when bodies appear to be culturally de-civilized, of what 'everyone else' is not: dedicated, controlled, disciplined, culturally and economically invested in health and self-responsible" (176). Certainly completing a triathlon requires a significant time and resource commitment, but does such a significant commitment really ameliorate the world by empowering others to do the same? I would argue that, much like the completion of a marathon as part of a "bucket-list," such demonstrations are not as enduring as those of the runner and cyclist who may at times have such aspirations, but ultimately are not moved by such objectives. I wonder if the more ameliorative route would be to convince the nonathlete to commit to a shorter distance—those more representative of the runner.

It is here that the representative nature of the running and cycling community may have its greatest effect. While athletes may have the spotlight in the competitive world, those competitions consist of only a fraction of their actual performance time. As noted by Hockey (2006), "the vast majority of running undertaken by these athletes is done during training runs, which far outweighs their involvement in racing" (184). In essence, where the athletes seek to be most visible, to overcome distance in short bouts of time in competitive settings, does not demonstrate the bulk of their focused efforts to others. In a similar way, joggers/riders do not train enough to have a visible presence in the endurance landscape.

The goals of the runners and cyclists, however, do not specifically include competitive glory although they do have a significant presence in the endurance community. It is due to their positioning within the overall endurance angle of vision that runners and cyclists are poised to best engage in the dialectical relationship with others. As Smith (2000) notes:

> People gain no particular kudos from their sporting performances as a mediocre badminton or squash player. However, since runners believe that the distances they cover in racing and training impress nonparticipants, their involvement is felt to deliver status, respect, and admiration to those who run at a nonelite level as well. (202)

## A RETURN TO GENIUS

As I noted at the outset of this chapter, in many ways Emerson's *Representative Men* is an examination of the existence of genius—of people who in their characteristics and actions answer questions that ordinary people do not even have the skill to ask. Perhaps we can say that runners and cyclists are the best representatives of endurance sport, but can we say that all runners and cyclists should be considered genius? Certainly not, especially if we hone in on Emerson's insistence that the amelioration of the world resides in the runners' and cyclists' ability to not only reveal specific aspects of nature but additionally empower "ordinary people" with the insight to reorient their lives for the betterment of the world. Yet in the case of endurance sport, who are the "ordinary people" who stand to benefit from such revelation?

I would suggest that the growing numbers of sedentary individuals throughout the world are dangerously close to defining the "ordinary" or familiar population. The United States' Center for Disease Control and Prevention (CDC) noted that 36 percent of all U.S. adults were rated as obese in the years 2011–2014 and all states had an obesity rating of 20 percent or higher in 2015 (www.cdc.gov/obesity/data/adult.html). The World Health Organization (WHO) also noted that worldwide obesity rates have more than doubled since 1980 (www.who.int/mediacentre/factsheets/fs311/en/). With the ongoing developments in technology, transportation, food production, and industrialization, humans simply do not have the vital need to move as much as they used to for their survival.[14] I am certainly not a Luddite, but the idea of moving for any purpose, or for no specific purpose at all, seems to be losing traction within world culture.

I suggest that the non-mover is becoming more and more the "ordinary." As such, I suggest that it is the quality of the interface between mover and non-mover where endurance sports genius resides. Genius can be found within the running and cycling representatives of endurance sport as those individuals who best demonstrate a commitment to Emerson's dialectical relationship with others. The genius in endurance sport dwells within the ability to ameliorate the world by getting others to see the value in, and ultimately participate in, movement and endurance activities. As I noted above, runners and cyclists move not primarily as a means to some external goal. Rather, they use their activities to reveal the inherent qualities of what appears to "ordinary" people as mundane, commonplace, and often unnecessary experiences. It is not principally about the miles and minutes, but rather about the conceptualization of those miles and minutes as deeply personal and meaningful experiences.

The trick is to transform those personal and meaningful experiences, those that are personally ameliorative, into something palatable for others. In some ways, runners and cyclists have to be like Napoleon, one of Emerson's "Great Men" who could carry "the power and affections of vast numbers" (Emerson, 1996, 129) as well as like Goethe, who Emerson described as exemplary of the notion that "all things are engaged in writing their history" and, furthermore, "that men are born to write" (Emerson, 1996, 151–152). Simply, I suggest that true genius in the endurance community is, in part, the ability to be a good storyteller. It is the ability to make descriptions of one's activities come alive to others—the sights, sounds, and feels of the run or the ride. It is the ability to package those stories empathetically so that the listener can see themselves in the runners' and cyclists' footsteps and pedal strokes. It is the ability to have the non-mover believe and internalize an "I can do that" attitude and then actually go out and ameliorate the world by doing it.

This is why the runner and cyclist are ultimately in the best position to represent the endurance community. Stories of the jogger and rider, such as those told by Wisnewski of the unpleasant obstacles of time and distance, are not good catalysts for a dialectical relationship between non-mover and mover. Similarly, stories from athletes driven by competitive fervor and significant mileage would most likely result in unrealistic expectations or thoughts of impossibility. Runners and cyclists are in the best place to have that dialectical interface with others. While there are no guarantees that such amelioration will be transposed from one to the other, a visibility and understanding of the endurance sports practice to a greater degree than the jogger and rider but valued beyond the accounting of minutes and miles aimed at competitive success positions runners and cyclists as potential geniuses. The genius resides in a similar place as Emerson's description of Plato, his representative of philosophy. "All my good is magnetic," he writes, "and I educated not by lessons, but by going about my business" (Emerson, 1996, 38). The genius of the runner and the cyclist is realized when they ameliorate the world through the activation of others.

In the end, representatives of endurance sport are those who reveal the nature of the world through their exposition and embrace of the qualities of time and distance experienced as runners and cyclists. Endurance sport genius is found in the movement away from egotistical practices and to the empowerment of others with the knowledge to reorient their lives for the betterment of the world. In essence, the best representative endurance athletes are the runners that actuate other runners and the cyclists that beget other cyclists.

## NOTES

1. Plato (428/427–424/423 BC), or "the philosopher," was an Ancient Greek philosopher who Emerson described as a "complete man who could apply to nature the whole scale of the senses, the understanding, and the reason" (Emerson, 1996,

27). Emanuel Swedenborg (1688–1772), or "the mystic," was a Swedish theologian who Emerson critiqued as someone who "fastened each natural object to a theologic notion" to the point that "nothing with him had the liberality of universal wisdom, but we are always in a church" (Emerson, 1996, 68, 75). Michel de Montaigne (1533–1592), or "the skeptic," was a significant philosopher during the French Renaissance and served as Emerson's representative of "wise limitation," "some condition between extremes," and "the fit person to occupy the ground of speculation" (Emerson, 1996, 92). William Shakespeare (1564–1616), or "the poet," was an English poet, playwright, and actor who had the "power of expression, or of transferring the inmost truth of things into music and verse" (Emerson, 1996, 122). Napoleon Bonaparte (1769–1821), or "the man of the world," was a French military and political leader in early seventeenth-century France and represents a man who could "carry with him the power and affections of vast numbers" and express "the tone of thought and belief" of the masses (Emerson, 1996, 129). Finally, Johann Wolfgang von Goethe (1749–1832), or "the writer," was a prolific German writer who, for Emerson, represented the "powers and duties of the scholar or writer" as well as the "intellectual works of the period" (Emerson, 1996, 156).

2. While overall participation in running and cycling activities remains high (see Outdoor Foundation, 2016), participation in competitive running events has declined (Bush, 2017).

3. See Loland's work for the development of an ecosophy of sport (Loland, 1996, 2001, 2006).

4. These categories are taken from Smith (1998). However, Smith only identified joggers, runners, and athletes using several intertwined criteria: pace, distance, weekly mileage, regularity, and commitment (182). I have added analogous cycling monikers of rider, cyclist, and athlete to his typology and will use them throughout the paper to describe the endurance bicycling community. Certainly, these categories are fluid when considering the variability within each criterion and when contextualized within one's life narrative.

5. To be clear, I have no metric that determines the exact point when a jogger becomes a runner or when a runner becomes an athlete. Ultimately that determination resides within the experiences of the performers and the perception of those performers by others. However, metrics of distance and time certainly apply in all cases.

6. Again, these categories are fluid. Certainly a jogger/rider could commit to a training program and eventually test the limits of human endurance, but on the way to that limit, they would no longer be joggers and riders. They would be runners or cyclists and eventually athletes.

7. As noted earlier, Smith (1998) uses the criteria of pace, distance, weekly mileage, regularity, and commitment (182) to categorize joggers, runners, and athletes. I would suggest that "dabblers" fundamentally lack regularity and commitment. This does not suggest that those professed and practicing "slow" runners, such as John "The Penguin" Bingham (www.johnbingham.com), are "dabblers." Clearly someone like this who has a webpage dedicated to running, including "The Penguin's 100 Day Challenge" that has the goal of moving intentionally for at least 30 minutes a day, no matter what speed, is not a "dabbler."

8. For example, see www.runnersworld.com/fun/who-is-the-greatest-runner-of-all-time for runners and www.active.com/cycling/articles/the-10-greatest-road-cyclists-of-all-time for cyclists.

9. If this were the case, *prima facie* "representatives" of the endurance community would include runners such as Steve Prefontaine, Paula Radcliffe, and Mo Farah and cyclists such as Eddy Merckx, Miguel Idurain, and Lance Armstrong, to name a few.

10. Emerson's "representative" of philosophy, Plato, would most likely point to his cave allegory and suggest that the jogger, rider, and athlete simply need to turn toward the light to realize the runners' and cyclists' experiential possibilities.

11. In contrast, if I were to complete a "speed workout" on the same stretch of beach the experience would be quite different. I would have "used" it primarily for the achievement of purposeful, goal-driven outcomes—like an "athlete."

12. raystown.org/allegrippis-trails

13. While elite athletes could be considered "giants" in a similar fashion to Emerson's "Great Men," this would also be in contrast to his "egalitarian proposition" as noted in Gura's critique.

14. See Heinrich's (2001) *Why We Run*, particularly chapter thirteen, "Evolution of Intelligent Running Ape People," for an interesting discussion as to how humans are evolutionarily programmed to be endurance athletes.

# REFERENCES

Anderson, D. (2001). Recovering humanity: Movement, sport, and nature. *Journal of the Philosophy of Sport*, 28(2), 140–150.

Armstrong, L. (2000). *It's not about the bike*. New York: Berkley.

Atkinson, M. (2008). Triathlon, suffering and exciting significance. *Leisure Studies*, 27(2), 165–180.

Brenkus, J. (2010). *The perfection point*. New York: Harper Collins.

Bush, S. (2017). U.S. road race trends. Running USA (on-line). www.runningusa.org/2017-us-road-race-trends.

Caesar, E. (2015). *Two hours: The quest to run the impossible marathon*. New York: Simon & Schuster.

Corbitt, T. (1998). A willingness to suffer. In G. Kislevitz (Ed.), *First marathons* (pp. 79–88). New York: Bantam Dell.

Coyle, D. (2009). *The talent code*. New York: Bantam Books.

Colvin, G. 2008. *Talent is overrated*. London: Portfolio.

Emerson, R.W. (1981). *The portable Emerson*. Bode, C. (Ed.). New York: Penguin Books.

Emerson, R.W. (1996). *Representative men*. Cambridge, MA: The Belknap Press of Harvard University Press.

Epstein, D. (2013). *The sports gene*. New York: Current.

Gladwell, M. (2008). *Outliers: The story of success*. New York: Little, Brown and Company.

Gura, P.F. (1977). Thoreau's Maine woods Indians: More representative men. *American Literature*, 49, 366–384.
Heinrich, B. (2001). *Why we run: A natural history*. New York: Harper Collins.
Hochstetler, D.R. (2003). Process and the sport experience. *Quest*, 55(3), 231–243.
Hockey, J. (2006). Sensing the run: The senses and distance running. *The Senses and Society*, 1(2), 183–201.
Hopsicker, P.M. (2010). Learning to ride a bike. In J. Ilundain-Agurruza and M.W. Austin (Eds.), *Cycling: Philosophy for everyone* (pp. 16–26). Malden, MA: Blackwell.
Hopsicker, P. (2011). In search of the 'sporting genius': Exploring the benchmarks to creative behavior in sporting activity. *Journal of the Philosophy of Sport*, 38(1), 113–127.
Hopsicker, P.M. and Hochstetler, D. (2014). Finding the 'me' in endurance sports: An apology for runners and joggers, cyclists and riders. *Kinesiology Review*, 3, 161–171.
Kalb, C. (2017). Genius. *National Geographic*, 231, PG #.
Lacerda, T. and Mumford, S. (2010). The genius in art and in sport: A contribution to the investigation of aesthetics of sport. *Journal of the Philosophy of Sport*, 37(2), 182–193.
Lockhart, B. (2010). Letters. *Running Times*. April (375), 8–9.
Loland, S. (1996). Outline of an ecosophy of sport. *Journal of the Philosophy of Sport*, 23, 70–90.
Loland, S. (2001). Record sports: An ecological critique and a reconstruction. *Journal of the Philosophy of Sport*, 28(2), 127–139.
Loland, S. (2006). Olympic sport and the ideal of sustainable development. *Journal of the Philosophy of Sport*, 33, 144–156.
McMahon, D.M. (2013). *Divine fury: A history of genius*. New York: Basic Books.
Outdoor Foundation. (2016). *Outdoor participation report 2016*. (www.outdoorfoundation.org). Washington, DC: The Outdoor Foundation.
Smith, S.L. (1998). Athletes, runners, and joggers: Participant-group dynamics in a sport of 'individuals'. *Sociology of Sport Journal*, 15, 174–192.
Smith, S.L. (2000). British nonelite road running and masculinity: A case of 'running repairs'? *Men and Masculinities*, 3(2), 187–208.
Wisnewski, J.J. (2007). The phenomenology of becoming a runner. In M.W. Austin (Ed.), *Running & philosophy* (pp. 35–43). Malden, MA: Blackwell.

*Chapter 6*

# Cooking up a Plan

## *Pragmatism and Training*

Pam R. Sailors and Cody D. Cash

Taken on its own, training is a vacuous concept. One does not simply train. One trains for something; one trains in certain ways—the concept has to be grounded in its intended outcome and process before it has any robust use in thought or activity. This is valuable to consider for every endurance athlete, as training regimens dictate fundamental aspects of their lives, and the selection of training plans is done with great care, ideally selecting the "right" one.

The pragmatist maxim advocated by Charles Sanders Peirce and William James—that one should clarify the contents of hypotheses and concepts by examining their "practical consequences"—is uniquely suited to evaluate the manner in which and by which endurance athletes scrutinize and ultimately utilize training plans. Abstract objective evaluations are of little value to racers; a given plan has value only insofar as it leads to an outcome desired by the trainee. This outcome is then used to assess the value or truth of the training plan for both the trainee and others who might wish to adopt the regimen.

In this chapter, we discuss James' view of truth and his claim that belief in something might make it so. We also consider Peirce's notion that inquiry is a struggle to replace doubt with settled belief and his four methods for settling belief. Then, we explain Lisa Heldke's contention that thinking about recipes and cooking can teach something about philosophical inquiry and theory-making. We outline how this view extends to training plans, allowing us better to evaluate them using the tools of pragmatism. At the same time, our examples of endurance athletes and their use of training plans may also function to enhance understanding of pragmatism.

## USE YOUR TRUTH WISELY

For William James, the basis of truth for a given concept or object is to be found in its practical usefulness. According to James, something has meaning and value due to the use(s) it affords an individual as s/he navigates the world. A stick of wood is, in fact, a baseball bat if it can be used to hit a baseball; a cup is different from a mere container if it can be used to drink from; even belief in a given religion is meaningful if that belief provides a direction for the actions and attitudes it allows one to adopt.

This practical shift is the hallmark of pragmatism because "use" inherently involves an inseparable relationship between subject and object; a relationship that requires all concepts and valuations of those concepts to be derived from real-world experience. At the core of James' "radical empiricism" was the notion that subject and object should not be considered wholly independent entities because they cannot *practically* be contemplated as such. To contemplate baseball bat-ness, cup-ness, godliness, goodness, or truth requires grounding the concept in first-person experience if there is ever to be hope of reaching a conclusion. This is where his famous squirrel-going-round-the-tree story from his (1907) lecture, "What Pragmatism Means," comes into play. As the story goes, James' friends were unable to reach a conclusion as to whether a man circling a squirrel who was also circling a tree can ever be said to have gone around the squirrel. One group wanted to say going around requires seeing all sides of the squirrel, which the man never would if he and the squirrel remained on opposite sides of the tree as they went round. The other group focused on the cardinal directions—if one travelled north, south, east, and west of the squirrel (which would occur even if the man and squirrel remained on opposite sides), then one could be said to have gone around it. The two conflicting camps of "to go round" were at an impasse that abstract reasoning could not resolve, as both seem to be rational definitions of the term. James' solution was simple: use them. Try the definitions out in the world, and whichever coheres best with experience and proves to be most widely applicable, without contradiction or disuse, is the one to adopt.

In this way, pragmatism for James is a method. Rather than taking a static stance about any truth or principle through reason alone, one should form a rational hypothesis and test it through reason *and* experience. Thus, James prescribes that we "try to interpret each notion by tracing its respective practical consequences," and ask, "[w]hat difference would it practically make to anyone if this notion rather than that notion were true?" (James 1978, 28). Once we have answered that question, we will find that: "Our conception of these effects, whether immediate or remote, is then for us the whole of our conception of the object, so far as that conception has positive significance at all" (James 1978, 29). The steadfast focus of the pragmatic method on practical consequences reframes inquiries of truth by what that truth accomplishes. Rather than treating truth as an abstracted, *a priori* state, it has cash value—the ability of a given object or concept to achieve certain ends: "Theories thus become instruments, not answers to enigmas, on which we can rest" (James 1978, 32).

However, the ability to achieve certain ends is ambiguous. It is dependent upon the subjective desires of the individual and the ability of the subject(s) to verify whether those ends have been achieved. And if there can be no one-to-one correspondence with absolute, objective truth, how can anything be successfully verified? In other words, if there is no capital "T" Truth to which one can refer or rely on, what is providing the verification? According to James, the verification comes from consistency and coherence with other beliefs:

> The true is whatever is opposite of whatever is instable, of whatever lying and unreliable, of whatever is unverifiable and unsupported, of whatever is inconsistent and contradictory, of whatever is artificial and eccentric, of whatever is unreal in the sense of being of no practical account. (James 1978, 214)

Imagine, for example, a runner considering competing in the early years of the Barkley Marathons. As an ultramarathon covering 100+ miles in the rugged Tennessee wilderness, with more than 50,000 feet of accumulated vertical climb, the race would have presented a novel experience for the runner as a race. Aside from the formidable challenges offered from the terrain and length, another unique feature is that it's not a race in the usual sense. Most "races" have the inherent assumption that competitors will finish, with the winner being the competitor who finishes first. The competitor who finishes first at the Barkley Marathons will also be crowned the winner, but there is no guarantee there will be a winner at all. It's not uncommon for the vast majority of competitors not to finish the race; some years, no one does. Thus, if the runner's experience had provided the foundation for the notion that all races begin with the expectation that at least one person will finish, it would have been difficult for that individual to believe the Barkley Marathons were a race. S/he might have chosen to investigate further by attending or attempting to complete the event, to determine if the Barkley Marathons should have been considered a race or just a challenge or some complicated form of public masochism (which might be true for all endurance sports). But in the meantime, the lack of coherence with other beliefs at least would have given the runner pause and reason to suspend the adoption of the new belief or "truth" about whether this event should have been considered a race. And if the runner chose not to investigate further, the event may never have been considered a race for him/her. In this case, truth is neither absolute nor infallible. Truth becomes a malleable property or attribute of a given concept or thing rather than an abstracted class it either does or does not fit into: "truth is *made*, just as health, wealth and strength are made, in the course of experience" (James 1978, 104).

This is not to say that truth must be decided or verified solely on the basis of the individual's experience, but it must be based on someone's experience, sometime and someplace. Individuals may trade on one another's truths—perhaps the runner asks others if they have ever participated in such events—in order to interpret novel situations or to consider affairs with which one has no direct experience, and in doing so may reach a high level of agreement among individuals. Yet, even when this occurs and there is a sort of stability of human exchange and communication, the reason for keeping the agreement or holding on to the shared truth is still based on its having been verified or having paid out for an individual, coupled with the belief that it will do so again in the future: "You accept my verification of one thing, I yours of another. We trade on each other's truth. But beliefs verified concretely by *somebody* are the posts of the whole superstructure" (James 1978, 100).

So, truth is made, fallible, and always born from individual experience, but why investigate it or adopt any truths at all? Just as Hume proclaimed reason to be the slave of the passions, James embraces the idea that one's truths, at bottom, are derived from one's passions and desires, claiming that "our non-intellectual nature *does* influence our convictions. There are passional tendencies and volitions which run before and others which come after belief, and it is only the latter that are too late for the fair" (James 1896, 334, emphasis added).

Importantly, one's desire for a truth to obtain can help bring that truth about. Wanting something to be true can affect how one will perceive the world and courses of action one might take, thus influencing the verification process itself. In "The Will to Believe," James (James 1896) describes how the question of whether another person likes you or not will be answered, in part, by the unjustified beliefs you hold beforehand. If you believe the person does like you, you might be more open to conversation with him/her, smile, make eye contact, etc. These actions might then lead to that person responding in kind, which would then verify the belief that s/he likes you. On the other hand, if you start with the belief that the other person does not like you, you might avoid conversation and eye contact, and generally behave in a way that contributes to the other person not liking you: "In truths dependent on our personal action, then, faith based on desire is certainly a lawful and possibly indispensible thing" (James 1986, 343). Thus, for James, truth is an attribute of a concept or thing determined by how successful it is in consistently serving the goals and desires of individuals, collectively and in isolation. Truth is fallible, shaped by subjectivity, and always has practical value. In short, it must be useful.

James derived his view of truth from the work of Charles Sanders Peirce, who created pragmatism only to distance himself later from what it had become. In fact, Peirce came to call his position "critical common-sensism" or "pragmaticism" to distinguish it from that of James, Schiller, and others, famously announcing that he

> finding his bantling "pragmatism" so promoted, feels that it is time to kiss his child good-bye and relinquish it to its higher destiny; while to serve the precise purpose of expressing the original definition, he begs to announce the birth of the world "pragmaticism," which is ugly enough to be safe from kidnappers. (Peirce 1955, 255)

While there are numerous differences between the positions of James and Peirce, the primary difference we wish to highlight is the contrast between James' seeming acceptance of the notion that individuals can create truth versus Peirce's insistence on the essential role of the community in determining belief.

According to Peirce, we are motivated to seek belief by the discomfort we feel when in doubt: "With the doubt . . . the struggle begins, and with the cessation of doubt it ends. Hence the sole object of inquiry is the settlement of opinion" (Peirce 1955, 10). There are four ways this inquiry may play out, or, in Peirce's terms, four methods of fixing belief. First, is the method whereby one decides what to believe and simply refuses to admit any further evidence. Peirce compares this to an ostrich burying its head in the sand. Perhaps more familiar today, social media allows us to surround ourselves with others who believe and experience life in the same way. Unlike the ostrich, humans are unlikely to remain satisfied by this approach because we are unlikely to be able to avoid opposing opinions:

> This method of fixing belief, which may be called the method of tenacity, will be unable to hold its ground in practice. The social impulse is against it. The man who adopts it will find that other men think differently from him, and it will be apt to occur to him, in some saner moment, that their opinions are quite as good as his own, and this will shake his confidence in his belief. (Peirce 1955, 12)

Authority, the second method of fixing belief, may be characterized as macro-tenacity. Instead of an individual establishing belief, it is the state that sets acceptable doctrines and prohibits any teaching of alternatives. This method may find some success, but will be defeated, again by the social impulse, as people recognize that divergent beliefs are taught by other states. Thus, Peirce says both "willful adherence to a belief, and the arbitrary forcing of it upon others" (Peirce 1955, 14) must be abandoned.

The third method fares no better, defeated in the end by the impulse that has sometimes occasioned it. Peirce calls this the *a priori* method and describes it as arising from the experience of doubt about existing beliefs. Communication with others raises doubt and then alleviates it by bringing diverse beliefs into harmony with what people approve:

> Systems of this sort have not usually rested upon any observed facts, at least not in any great degree. They have been chiefly adopted because their fundamental propositions seemed "agreeable to reason." This is an apt expression; it does not mean that which agrees with experience, but that which we find ourselves inclined to believe. (Peirce 1955, 15)

For example, Descartes, led by doubt, concluded that he could accept only those beliefs he clearly and distinctly perceived. Peirce suggests this method cannot work because people will eventually come to doubt beliefs that are not caused by facts drawn from experience.

The methods of tenacity, authority, and *a priori* have in common an origin in human thought. The fourth method—that of science—differs in that it accepts beliefs only if they are determined not by what anyone thinks, but by the perception of external objects, what Peirce calls "Real" things. Hence, "by taking advantage of the laws of perception, we can ascertain by reasoning how things really and truly are; and any man, if he have sufficient experience and he reason enough about it, will be led to the one True conclusion" (Peirce 1955, 19). What is being advocated here is beginning with the stimulus of doubt, following the scientific method of testing hypotheses, and concluding with the settlement of opinion.

With this basic sketch of the theoretical commitments of James and Peirce in place, we move to application. Rather than apply the pragmatic method directly from what's been discussed, we utilize an analogy provided by Lisa Heldke, who suggests we craft truth-seeking theories in much the same way we make and use cooking recipes, with a greater emphasis on subjective goals than infallible and immutable truths. This analogy is particularly helpful for our purposes because endurance sport training plans are often treated in the same way as recipes—as rigid gospel by those new to the endeavor and as a customizable base for those with a good deal of experience.

## THE PRAGMATIC RECIPE FOR TRAINING PLANS

In "Recipes for Theory Making" (1988), Lisa Heldke draws primarily on the work of John Dewey to offer a position she called the "coresponsible" option. This position is motivated by Heldke's belief that both foundationalism and relativism are flawed frameworks. Foundationalism, in its insistence that there exist universally consistent *a priori* principles, views difference as a lack of knowledge. As soon as we discover these principles, all differences will be eliminated by the one Truth. According to this model, all roads do not lead to Rome; instead there is only one road, one method, which is capable of approaching the Truth. Further, it is assumed that arriving in Rome is the only goal worthy of pursuit. All claims that other roads and other destinations might be legitimate are denied. Differences are taken to be evidence of a lack of understanding as there is only one theory and one method.

Relativism, Heldke contends, is equally flawed in its insistence that one may legitimately choose to follow any path on the way to any destination. The route chosen can never be criticized because all routes are equally legitimate. Thus, there is no limit to the number of theories that may be chosen and no possibility of criticizing the theories of others.

Heldke is not satisfied by either foundationalism or relativism because she is convinced that an examination of the actual world shows that it is neither plausible to claim, with the foundationalist, that respect for differences only exhibits a lack of understanding, nor plausible to claim, with the relativist, that all difference should be respected. We need an alternative position that will allow us to honor differences in attitudes without issuing a blanket approval of all attitudes and actions. Heldke's candidate for this median position is her Coresponsible Option.

The term "coresponsible" is meant to point to the fact that inquiry is characterized as taking place in an environment in which we are involved in relationships both with other inquirers and with that about which we are inquiring. In order for our inquiry to be successful, the environment must be one of cooperation and communication. Instead of the traditional view which holds that there is a radical dichotomy between subject and object, Heldke proposes that

> we think of inquiry as a communal activity, that we emphasize the relationships that obtain between inquirers and inquired. In the words of John Dewey, inquiry is "... the correspondence of two people [or things] who 'correspond' in order to modify one's own ideas, intents, and acts". (Heldke 1988, 17)

Subject and object are not seen as radically separate entities that are incapable of interacting in a way that affects each of them. Instead the relationship is reciprocal; subject and object mutually affect and alter each other in a transactional process.

Heldke's stance is also supported by the claims of Charles Peirce. Peirce is adamant in his insistence that no individual can discover truth without interaction with other inquirers and with reality itself. Successful inquiry is a process which necessarily involves cooperation and communication between inquirers; in this interaction, reality itself is discovered. Thus, Peirce says:

> The real, then, is that which, sooner or later, information and reasoning would finally result in, and which is therefore independent of the vagaries of me and you. Thus, the very origin of the conception of reality shows that this conception essentially involves the notion of a COMMUNITY, without definite limits, and capable of a definite increase of knowledge. (Peirce 1955, 247)

William James also stresses the relational character of inquiry with his assertion that inquiry is "a rich and active commerce . . . between particular thoughts of ours, and the great universe of other experiences in which they play their parts and have their uses" (James 1978, 39).

Heldke uses the word "option" to stress that she is offering one way, but not the only possible way, to approach theory. Here she is true to the spirit of fallibilism adopted by all the pragmatists as well as to their instrumentalist view of theories. Advocating the attitude of fallibilism, Peirce says that "any scientific proposition whatever is always liable to be refuted and dropped at short notice" (Peirce 1955, 54) because "we cannot in any way reach perfect certitude nor exactitude" (Peirce 1955, 58). This also parallels James' claim that theories should be thought of as instruments rather than answers to enigmas. It may also bring to mind the historical refutation and abandonment of the use of substances, like heroin and strychnine, that athletes once believed enhanced performance (Hoberman 2007). Thus, in her explanation of the name of her position, Heldke perfectly parallels the thought of the early pragmatists.

The spirit embodied by Heldke's Coresponsible Option is clear; now the content will be examined. Heldke uses the relationship of recipes and cooking as a model to describe the construction and implementation of theory through the process of inquiry. She considers five aspects of recipes and cooking, showing that the processes of inquiry are the same as the processes of recipe use in each case. At each stage of her analysis, Heldke's position remains consistent with pragmatism.

The first characteristic of recipe making that Heldke notes is that there are a variety of reasons why cooks develop new recipes and experiment with modifications of existing recipes. The cook may be motivated by a lack of money, an urge for novelty, or dietary restraints. The amount of experimenting that one does is determined (or at least influenced) by the particular goal one wants to reach. This fact, when applied to theory, strongly suggests that the foundationalist is incorrect to claim that there is only one Truth which we all want to pursue. Instead, "theories, like recipes, are most usefully thought of as tools we use to do things" (Heldke 1988, 21). Just as we need different tools to accomplish different tasks, we need different theories in order to successfully maneuver our way through the world.

Instead of seeing theories as something that will result in one specific product, Heldke suggests that we see the goal, or product of theorizing as the practical use we make of the theory in our relationships in, and to, the world. In a footnote, Heldke notes:

> There still seems to be a troubling disparity between cooking and theorizing, however, because it seems that cooking produces food a lot more often than theories produce practical consequences in one's life in the world. Precisely. I think this is a failure of theorizing. (Heldke 1988, 29)

This comment puts Heldke squarely within the pragmatist camp as it echoes both Peirce and James. Peirce offers the following principle for attaining complete clarity: "Consider what effects that might conceivably have practical bearing you conceive the object of your conception to have. Then your conception of those effects is the WHOLE of your conception of the object" (Peirce 1955, 259). Heldke's criticism is also supported by James' claim that "ideas (which themselves are about parts of our experience) become true just in so far as they help us to get into satisfactory relations with other parts of our experience" (James 1978, 34).

Heldke acknowledges that few cooks engage in dramatic experimentation because few cooks have sufficient knowledge of the properties of the foods with which they cook. Most cooks are deterred from gaining this knowledge because it is only attained after long and careful study. However, if one *is* willing to make the effort, the result is of great benefit as it allows one to be creative and flexible. This fact is also applicable to theorizing. Heldke draws the connection this way:

> It's relatively easy to take up a theory, wholecloth, and use it. But to do so is to run the heavy risk of being irrelevant, harmful, or destructive. To do useful theory, I think it is necessary to explore and experiment, to know extremely well the things with which you're inquiring. (Heldke 1988, 22)

If my theory does not take into account the relations you have with the rest of the world, then my theory will be no more successful than a recipe that doesn't take altitude into account when giving instructions for baking time.

This characteristic is also evident in endurance sport training plans. When searching for and selecting a plan, the critical question is, "What will I achieve by following this plan?" Some plans will tout an objective outcome based on finish time ("Break 3:00 Marathon Plan"), training duration ("12 Week Olympic Triathlon Training Plan"), or training frequency ("4 Days/Week Marathon Training Plan"), while others are more overtly subjective ("A Plan for a Marathon PR"). Yet all have the same basic conditional tied to their expected outcomes: if I follow this plan, then I will be able to complete this race (possibly within a certain time). As with the squirrel going around the tree story, James's method to solving the dilemma of choosing the correct plan would be to use them and see which is most widely applicable without disuse or contradiction. For example, if the "Break 3:00 Marathon Plan" is followed precisely and leads to a 3:20 finish time, it's not a good or truthful plan; whereas if it does lead to one or many races under the three-hour mark, it should be considered good and truthful.

Just as Heldke is suggesting with recipes and theories, training plans should not be seen as resulting in one specific product or outcome for all. If a plan were described as "The BEST triathlon plan" it would be a very poorly named plan. Best in what way? Best for guaranteeing a certain time? Best for new competitors? Best for improving cycling technique and time? "Best" is ambiguous and only gains practical meaning through an individual's current athletic prowess and desired goal. Thus, to say X is the best plan, or the best plan at achieving Y, is to claim a singular, objective truth. And just as there is more than one way to cook a chicken, there is more than one way to train for a triathlon. The more accurate way to describe a plan would be to say it is the best plan *for me* to complete a triathlon, or *for me* to improve on the cycling portion. This eliminates the capital "T" truth of the plan while also grounding its value in the relationships it helps an athlete create in, and to, the world. In this way, a given plan only becomes useful and meaningful for athletes when evaluated under a more subjective lens.

The second characteristic of recipes to which Heldke points is that many more of them are collected and exchanged by cooks than are actually used. Many people read recipes and imagine what it might be like to prepare them without any serious intent to implement them. It is often the case, however, that a new recipe suggests to the mind of the reader possibilities for modifications of old recipes. Perhaps a new ingredient is discovered that might be useful for altering the taste or nutritional value of a favorite dish. This fact about the use of recipes suggests a new way to view theories:

> I think of philosophical theorizing as collecting, trading, developing, using, adapting and discarding recipes/theories. I collect ideas from various sources. Some of them I try—and some of these I keep and modify for use again. Others I talk and think about, the way I talk about what a recipe might taste like and how long it might take to prepare. They don't become a part of my theoretical/ practical life, but hover in the wings, waiting for a situation in which they might be useful. (Heldke 1988, 22)

Good theories will draw from a variety of sources just as good cooks will draw from a variety of recipes.

The use of training plans, like recipes, is rarely a one-time event for an athlete or cook and rarely is a plan completed unaltered. It is possible there are people who devote themselves to a single sport and training plan during their lifetimes and never deviate from the parameters, but such individuals are definitely not the norm. This is because we are complex creatures who adopt these plans for different reasons at different times in our lives hoping for a wide range of outcomes.

If, for example, a first-time marathon runner once competed in middle distance races, she might believe that plans incorporating a certain amount of speed work on the track will work best because that type of training has paid dividends in the past. In this case, her unique past and situation affect the manner in which she first approaches an endurance sport training plan. This is similar to recipes in that someone will not even consider a recipe calling for cooking over an open flame if electric heat is the only option—in order for the recipe to be considered a viable option, it must build upon methods and utensils with which the cook is familiar or can learn to use. And once the cook or runner becomes comfortable with the methods and outcomes of the recipe or plan, creativity and community come into play.

Unlike months-long training plans, almost any recipe can be tried in a few hours or less. Once tested, one can choose to keep it as is, add a little more salt, cook longer, alter ingredients, etc., in a short time with minimal risk. (If you make a disgusting batch of cookies by substituting mayonnaise for shortening, oh well. A much tastier batch can be created within the hour.) Endurance sport training plans can't be tested in the same way because the stakes are too high and the factors in play over the many weeks and months of the plan are too many. This creates a bit of a challenge when considering the highly variegated biases athletes already possess when evaluating training plans. The solution is what Heldke and the pragmatists suggest: we turn to the community to collect and trade knowledge. A man living in the Rocky Mountains might ask other mountain marathoners what plans worked best for them and if and how they altered them to work when training at altitude. A runner who can only commit to running four times a week will find plans that fit that criteria and then look up reviews from those who have attempted them to determine which one to choose. And a woman who has completed more than one marathon will compare her past experience in both training and the races with the experiences of others to determine which plan or plans to parse and combine to create a plan suited to her own specific goals and situation.

That the way recipes are created and exchanged exhibits some freedom of choice is the third characteristic of recipes/cooking cited by Heldke. There is no one way to prepare food and there is no one food that all cooks must choose to prepare. A recipe is a suggestion that we may accept, modify, or refuse. We may think of theory in the same way. A theory is a suggestion of a goal and a way to reach that goal. Though a person is likely to show some positive bias toward authors whose previous theories have proven to be useful to him/her, each new theory from that author will still be tested and there is no absolutist claim about the project or the theory. Even if one tends to examine theories born from a certain individual or along similar lines of thought, other theories may work just as well or better than the one being suggested. Thus, the foundationalist horn of the dilemma is avoided.

This model also avoids the relativistic horn of the dilemma because our choices are not unlimited. All recipes have their breaking point beyond which they may not be altered. Some allow less modification than others; push these recipes beyond their breaking point and their integrity is lost. If, for example, you choose to prepare squash casserole, you cannot choose to leave out the squash. Your choice of ingredients is limited by your choice of recipes. Likewise, missing one day of running will not ruin an entire triathlon training plan; cutting out running altogether would probably undermine the whole endeavor. Linking this to theory, Heldke says even our original choice of a theory is influenced by our particular concerns. Once a theory is chosen, that theory further limits our choices of modifications. Each theory, like each recipe, has its breaking point beyond which it ceases to be the same theory.

Pulling these elements together to illustrate how theory making can avoid both absolutism and relativism, Heldke says:

> I've been drawing a picture of nested concerns-and-suggestions; I've suggested that selecting a particular moral stance might restrict the recipes I use, while selecting a particular recipe might restrict the ingredients and methods I use to execute it. At no level have I labelled something as "imperative," because in the strongest sense of the word, *nothing* is imperative. (Heldke 1988, 25)

Even the rules that we may think of as absolute rest on some prior choices. But, at all points of our choosing, the choices we make are limited to some degree by our projects and by our conceptualizations of the world. Does this third claim about recipe/theory square with pragmatism? It seems so.

Heldke's view of the presentation of a recipe/theory as a suggestion which may be refused echoes Peirce's introduction of his own work. He says he offers the fruits of his exploration, not as an imperative, but in the hope that others might benefit from what he has found useful. He "will suggest certain ideas and certain reasons for holding them true; but then, if you accept them, it must be because you like [his] reasons, and the responsibility lies with you" (Peirce 1955, 3). He refuses to issue an absolute assertion because, as he later argues, absolute assertion dangerously "blocks the way of inquiry" (Peirce 1955, 54). When theories are offered as suggestions rather than imperatives, we are free to choose the theory that is most useful to our chosen projects.

A look at the work of James provides support for Heldke's claim that choice is involved even in what we often take to be absolutely foundational principles. Choice of theory is influenced by the nature of the individual: "Temperaments with their cravings and refusals do determine [people] in their philosophies and always will" (James 1978, 24). Yet, as James points out, the context-specific nature of our choice of theories does not plunge us into relativism because our choices must bear fruit in the concrete world. Pragmatism avoids relativism because:

> You must bring out of each word its practical cash-value, set it at work within the stream of your experience. It appears less as a solution, then, than as a program for more work, and particularly as an indication of the ways in which existing realties may be *changed*. (James 1978, 31–32)

A recipe/theory is neither absolute nor relativistic because it must bear fruitful consequences in actual use, and because it must be referred back to our experience to suggest new ways of conceptualizing.

Even though training plans appear to be meticulously prescriptive, there are opportunities even here for choice and creativity within the structure. Scott Tinley, one of the pioneers of the sport of triathlon, acknowledges the freedom of choice within limits, noting:

Our season was long, March to October, or year-round if you wanted to race in the Southern Hemisphere during the winter. And during the eight-month season were distinct phases within each month, each week, each workout, and each race. Even though there were large similarities in training across each micro- and macro-cycle, there was enough creative opportunity to keep things new and fresh, so that the same damn 5,000-yard pool workout you had done fifty times before could still seem novel. It is like painting in oil on a twelve-by-fourteen-inch canvas: The size and medium are the same, but the possibilities are limitless (Tinley 2003, 134–135).

Similarly, Matt Fitzgerald's extended account of the 1989 Ironman Triathlon in Kona pointed out that "The details of their training methods are surprisingly varied, which suggests that these details are not terribly important. . . . 'The ingredients to proper training aren't a secret, and no one has the proper recipe anyway,' Mark [Allen] said early in his career" (Fitzgerald 2011, 228). No one has *the* proper recipe because there is no one proper recipe. Instead there are possible options, among which one is free to choose depending on one's tastes, interests, experience, and abilities.

Heldke has suggested that recipes/theories, while flexible, have certain limits beyond which they cannot be pushed. She has also offered the view that each of us must assess the usefulness of a particular recipe/theory for our lives. The fourth characteristic feature of recipes which she presents is that we can make these determinations only if we have adequate knowledge of the practice and the motives of those who offer the recipes to us. I must know something about the source of the recipe in order to determine why the specific instructions have been given. One may be told that using a particular type of cheese is necessary, but this instruction may merely be a reflection of the taste of the person who suggests the recipe. What sounds like an imperative may actually be only a personal preference. In order to know which is the case, one must have knowledge of the person who is the source of the recipe.

If we look at theories in the same light, we see that the usefulness and flexibility of a theory can only be assessed if we have sufficient knowledge of the motives of the person who offers the theory. By substituting "theory" for "recipe" in the following passage from Heldke, the point is made obvious:

> In general, when I receive a [theory], the more I know about the [theory] giver, the better the position I'll be I to assess the relevance *for me* of their instructions. And. When I'm in the position of giving out [theories], the more I take into account my recipient, the more I attempt to give information that is sensitive to their level of experience, the better off my recipient will be. (Heldke 1988, 26)

It may become clear to us, when we examine the motives of the theory giver, that the theory is much more flexible than it sounds. Statements that are issued as imperatives may really only be reflections of the personal preferences of the theory giver. We may also find that the theory is so tightly bound up in the motives of the giver that it cannot be accepted without also accepting those motives. Further, knowledge of the one to whom we suggest theories should have an influence on how we present our theories. We must know the other in order to know what common ground we might stand upon to persuade the other that our theory is worthwhile.

When applying this element to training plans, it is clear that the motives of the provider of the plan matter. The provider who is motivated by a desire to make a profit, so charging a fee for the provision of information, will likely offer something very different from the provider who is motivated only by a desire to pass on information that will help someone achieve a goal. The history of the sport of triathlon offers examples of providers with different motives:

> Around the . . . mid-1990s, the geeks invaded. A new wave of coaches came along and published influential books detailing training formulas that required a master's degree to understand and apply. These systems, with their cycles and phases and zones, were later complemented by computer programs that made the correct way to train even more dazzlingly complicated. There are now well-paid experts who specialize in adjusting the positioning of triathletes on their bikes. That's it. And, of course, there are other experts who do nothing but videotape athletes running and teach them how to run more correctly. (Fitzgerald 2011, 229–230)

This works in the opposite direction as well, regarding the motives of the recipient of the plan. The plan I would suggest for someone whose goal is to finish a marathon would be very different from the plan for someone whose goal is to break four hours. The plan for someone who is willing to run six days a week and do speedwork is different from someone who will run only four days a week with no speedwork. The usefulness of a plan can't be assessed without adequate knowledge of the motives of those involved in creating and executing that plan.

The final characteristic feature of recipes suggested by Heldke concerns the fact that recipes sometimes fail. Heldke believes that the failure, which may be the result of any number of causes, can be prevented by what she calls "thoughtful practice" (Heldke 1988, 27). Whether the problem is with the recipe or with the one who tries to utilize it, the failure can only be overcome by reflecting upon ways in which the practice can be fruitfully altered. To do so requires that we view the process as one which involves reciprocal relationships. The cook participates in a relationship with the ingredients and with the one who provided the recipe. Thoughtful practice corrects failures by recognizing these relationships and attempting to gain more information about the ones with whom we are in relation. Maybe the bread doesn't rise because I lacked knowledge of how it should be kneaded. Perhaps the cake fell because an ingredient was left out of the recipe someone gave me.

Heldke's application of this feature to theory contains a strong criticism of absolutism. Heldke explains:

> It won't do to treat theorizing as an activity in which I, the disinterested, semi-omniscient theory creator unveil a set of universally-applicable laws about a bunch of mute, lifeless Stuff of the Universe. Nor is it useful to think that I, the theory recipient, can simply take up someone else's theory as is, follow its unambiguous, universally-applicable instructions, and unproblematically apply it to the "same" phenomena they were exploring. (Heldke 1988, 28)

Only thoughtful practice can prevent theory-failure, and thoughtful practice requires us to recognize that we are in reciprocal relationships even with what we might be tempted to see as the "lifeless Stuff of the Universe." I take Heldke's use of scare quotes around "same" to indicate that the phenomena of the universe are, to some extent, different for each of us because each of us has a unique relationship with these phenomena. Thus, it is illegitimate to claim that any theory is universally and absolutely true.

Heldke's position here is easily supported by the words of the early pragmatists. Peirce, for example, claims that "there are three things to which we can never hope to attain by reasoning, namely, absolute certainty, absolute exactitude, absolute universality" (Peirce 1955, 56). This means that nothing bars the creation of, and experimentation with, theories. We are not completely free in our methods, but we are free in our attempt to develop theories that will reflect our relationships with the world. Peirce says:

> It is better to be methodical in our investigations, and to consider the economics of research, yet there is no positive sin against logic in *trying* any theory which may come into our heads, so long as it is adopted in such a sense as to permit the investigation to go on unimpeded and undiscouraged. (Peirce 1955, 54)

Heldke's claim that there is no universal semi-omniscient viewpoint from which one can issue forth theories may be read as a restatement of Peirce's position on the freedom we have to choose among existing theories and to create new ones.

James's essay on "The Moral Philosopher and the Moral Life" may also be seen as confirmation of Heldke's claim. James begins his essay with the declaration that "there is no such thing as an ethical philosophy dogmatically made up in advance" (James 1979, 184). Even *with* experience, it is impossible to formulate a theory that will apply to all people in all situations:

> For every real dilemma is in literal strictness a unique situation; and the exact combination of ideals realized and ideals disappointed which each decision creates is always a universe without a precedent, and for which no previous rule exists. (James 1979, 209)

This is just what Heldke has claimed. That is, no theory will equally and problematically apply to all situations because none of us experiences exactly the same phenomena. Further, any theory that is suggested may provide a useful guide to our unique situation, but it cannot issue an imperative (or "rule," in James's terms) that can fruitfully be followed in any and all experiences. In fact, this is true for the use of the cooking analogy as well; it may not be useful in analyzing all practices.

This is equally the case for training plans. In fact, in the early days of the triathlon, there were no training plans at all: "There was no blueprint on how to train. No coaches, camps, clinics, videos, or how-to manuals. It was all trial and error. And a ton of hard work" (Tinley 2003, 62). In retrospect, there was perhaps too much hard work:

> Certainly we erred on the side of too much distance. At one point . . . Scott Molina suggested that we combine the average weekly workouts of professional cyclists (400–500 miles), collegiate swimmers (20,000 yards), and Olympic marathoners (80–90 miles). And for a period . . . between 1982 and 1985, that is what we aimed for and came close. (Scott Tinley 2016, email to author)

This looking back and assessing what went wrong and how it might be prevented in the future, this trial and error, can be characterized as an application of Heldke's "thoughtful practice." In addition to over-training, athletes might fall short of their goals because the plan didn't match their level of ability, or recovery needs, or simply because of bad weather or a crowded field on race day. Thus, training plans, like recipes, sometimes fail to produce the desired product/outcome, but such failures can be illuminative with reflection on the relationships between athlete and the elements.

So, how ought we to evaluate the "Truth" of training plans? Given the preceding analysis, we suggest that asking the question is misguided. There is no practical value in pursuing the objective Truth of training plans. The more valuable pursuit is in testing and honing training plans. Rather than seeking the "right" plan(s), athletes benefit more by selecting the plan or plans they can best adopt and adapt—the plans that build on their past experience, available training time, training location, etc. The goal is not a plan that is right in an objective sense. Rather, the goal is a plan that works subjectively and allows the individual athlete to achieve his or her unique goals. We can no more make a comparative judgment of the infallible, immutable truth of differing training plans than we can about the truth of differing recipes for pies.

## REFERENCES

Fitzgerald, Matt. 2011. *Iron War: Dave Scott, Mark Allen and the Greatest Race Ever Run*. Boulder, CO: Velo Press.

Heldke, Lisa. 1988. "Recipes for Theory Making." *Hypatia: A Journal of Feminist Philosophy* 3(2): 15–29.

Hoberman, John. 2007. "Listening to Steroids." In *Ethics in Sport* 2nd edition, edited by William J. Morgan. Champaign, IL: Human Kinetics: 235–243.

James, William. 1896. "The Will to Believe." *The New World* 5: 327–347.

James, William. 1907. *Pragmatism: A New Name for Some Old Ways of Thinking*. http://www.gutenberg.org/files/5116/5116-h/5116-h.htm#link2H_4_0004

James, William. 1978. *Pragmatism and the Meaning of Truth*. Cambridge: Harvard University Press.

James, William. 1979. "The Moral Philosopher and the Moral Life." In *The Will to Believe and Other Essays in Popular Philosophy*, edited by Frederick Burkhardt, Fredson Bowers, and Ignas K. Skrupskelis (Eds.), Cambridge: Harvard University Press.

Peirce, Charles Sanders. 1955. *Philosophical Writings of Peirce*, edited by Justus Buchler. New York: Dover Publications.

Tinley, Scott. 2003. *Racing the Sunset: An Athlete's Quest for Life after Sport*. Guilford, CT: Lyons Press.

*Chapter 7*

# Dewey Goes the Distance

## Situated Habit and Ultraendurance Sports[1]

Jesús Ilundáin-Agurruza, Shaun Gallagher,
Daniel D. Hutto, and Kaarina Beam

### SIZING UP THE CHALLENGE: INTRODUCTION

Extraordinary open water swimmer Lynn Cox (2014) describes her experience when, as a 14-year-old, she did a 10-mile training swim in choppy seas off the coast of Santa Barbara, California, in 55F degree waters without wetsuit:

> I was working hard, enjoying it, drawing from every experience, learning how to feel the rhythm of the ocean, hear the tempo of the waves, and dance with the water using my balance, my strength, and all my senses. The waves grew louder and stronger. I improvised, adjusted the pitch of my hand, changed the rate of my strokes, and pressed my head deeper into the water so I could move through the waves instead of using more energy to bounce up and over them. (35)

We will return to this swim later. For now, it is suitable to highlight Cox's extraordinary exploits in long-distance swimming. Besides breaking the English Channel Crossing's absolute world record for both men and women when she was 15, she has done a number of first-ever traverses in some of the most arduous and coldest waters in the world, including a 12-hour crossing of the Cook Strait between the North and South Islands of New Zealand, and a mile-long 25-minute swim in Antarctica's 32F waters.

Cox exemplifies the kinds of sports and sportspersons at the center of this chapter: ultraendurance. As the prefix indicates, such sports take the notion of endurance to extremes (this does not *necessarily* mean that longer is harder or more difficult athletically). This increment marks quantitative amplification and deeply qualitative experiential changes that run the full gamut, from painfully gained existential epiphanies to socially extended cognitive facets. Others have drawn interesting philosophical lessons from endurance sports (Hochstetler and Hopsicker, 2012; 2016), but the severe efforts of the ultra dimension offer a unique window into a notion of performance that finds its raison d'être not in getting to the limit but in pushing beyond. Some (Dahl, 2016) stipulate a 6-hour mark for ultraendurance events, but instead of devising an always controversial definition, we offer a number of examples that showcase a wide range of ultra events.

Perhaps, the iconic event for ultraendurance sports is triathlon's Ironman competitions and their consecutive 2.5-mile swim, 112 miles of cycling, and marathon run. Then again, in the ultra world this looks amateurish when compared to events built on iterations of daily Ironman distances that add up to a Deca-Ironman (10 in 10 days), a triple-deca (30 in 30), or Ricardo Abad's record of 100 Ironman in one year (Abad, 2017). Ultrarunning is one of the most common. With races of 50, 100, 200 miles, and longer, it makes marathons seem but a warm-up lap. Other variations add daily marathons in consecutive days. Again, Abad holds the record with an astonishing 607 marathons in as many days. Closely related, adventure racing includes navigation and teamwork skills in events that last from eight hours to several weeks. Returning to the water, in standup paddling endurance events contestants paddle for hundreds of miles. Chris Bertish paddled 4,000 miles across the Atlantic Ocean in 93 days in 2017. Certainly, ultracycling events are paradigmatic ultra sports. The flagship events are the Race Across America (RAAM) 3,000-mile contest from the U.S. West to its East coast, and the tougher unsupported 4,300-mile Trans AM version. Mountaineering, with its protracted sorties and sustained efforts to summit, certainly qualifies. Other seemingly less athletically ultra sports can be as grueling and demanding on *all* levels, for example, offshore sailing or endurance motorized sports.

Defying common sense and a modicum of reasonableness, ultra sports are becoming more popular, with increasing numbers of competitors, events, and a growing list of activities. For instance, in 2014, in the United States alone, over 76,000 people participated in ultra-marathons that ranged from 50 to 200 miles (Barzilay, 2016). Perhaps the true litmus test of popularity is that the ultra phenomenon has attracted the attention of academia: 2017 marks the fourth edition of the annual international congress of *Medicine & Science in Ultra-Endurance Sports*.[2]

This chapter will explore the "ultra dimension" in relation to a situated approach to cognition and a pragmatist of renown, John Dewey. Given his temperament, William James would seem the ideal fit. He unapologetically embraced the strenuous life to the point that neopragmatist Richard Shusterman (2008) considers that James may have died prematurely on account of his exertions. But, it befalls on the more sedate Dewey to be our guide into the realm of the "Plus Ultra." His ideas afford particularly rich insights for these exuberant explorations into exaggeration. Dewey's opus, with over 300 published works and reams of collected unpublished writings, speaks of indefatigable efforts at the desk. More apropos is his commitment to a holistic view of human nature that seamlessly aligns with what today are called situated and enactive stances (Gallagher, 2009). These fall within the broader category of embodied cognition, whose origins are often attributed to Varela, Thompson and Rosch (1991). Simply put, the idea is that cognition arises from the interaction between organisms and environment rather than from the processing of abstract symbols, as philosophical orthodoxy would have it.

We can condense the versatility and applicability of Dewey's ideas to ultraendurance sports as a nurturing of skill through an "ethos of situated and dynamic habit." The remainder of the chapter lays out the rich details of this notion. The following list enumerates, in order of discussion, key Deweyan conceptual waypoints that signaly structure this inquiry: situatedness, body-mind, dynamic habit, deliberation, means/ends relation, self-discovery (flourishing), and social cognition. Other notable Deweyan notions, for example, "experience" or his "principle of continuity," are incorporated as pertinent. Along the way, ultraendurance standouts like Cox, skyrunner Kilian Jornet Burgada, novelist and runner Haruki Murakami, and sailor Ellen MacArthur among others will join this inquiry.

## GOING IN FOR THE LONG HAUL: SITUATED COGNITION AND AN ENACTIVE BODY-MIND

A preliminary discussion of the traditionally mainstream computational and representational stance (CRS) helps contextualize a situated and enactive model of cognition and skills. CRS views cognition in terms of information processing where such information is theorized as manipulation of abstract symbols with representational content that somehow mirrors the world. Put differently, semantic content realizes and individuates computational processes and states (at least partially). According to CRS, such content is necessary for sophisticated thought and action. The philosophical understanding of mental representation is cashed out in terms of truth or accuracy conditions of satisfaction. Simply and somewhat crudely illustrated, on that first ocean swim, Cox's performance was shaped by Cox forming and processing representations of waves, currents, and teammates in relation to her own position. That is, she was internally and symbolically representing what her mental states were about: relevant hydrodynamics, location, her own body. CRS is a dualistic approach: the mental symbols stand for pertinent features of the world. This form of dualism splits language and reality, mind and body, and individual and society (Bredo, 1994).

In contrast, the *situated and enactive account* (SEA) is a fluid and pluralist approach. Along with Dewey, it disavows computational processes and mental representation in lieu of direct, dynamical, and coevolving interactions between organisms and environments (Gallagher, 2017). As Eric Bredo (1994) explains,

> Just as an evolutionary biologist might focus on the coevolution of horses and grasses, seeing how each changed the other in a series of interactional cycles (Bateson, 1972), so Dewey focused on "doings and underdoings," which reciprocally change the character or structure of both person and environment, creating a joint history of development. (24)

This mutual influence needs to be emphasized, as it is not a mere juxtaposition but a holistic phenomenon. Richard Lally (2012) explains, "Within the pragmatic conception, all human action involved a transaction with the environment" (177).[3] Others, such as phenomenologist José Ortega y Gasset (2008), influenced by biologist Jacob von Uexküll (2010), highlighted such interaction, but in Dewey this is the keystone to his system of thought. The coupled transaction of organism *and* environment (such that the explanatory unit is "organism-environment") can be seen as an expression of Dewey's "principle of continuity":

> The primary postulate of a naturalistic theory of logic is continuity of the lower (less complex) and the higher (more complex) activities and forms . . . The idea of continuity . . . precludes reduction of the 'higher' to the "lower" just as it precludes complete breaks and gaps . . . what *is* excluded by the postulate of continuity is the appearance upon the scene of a totally new outside force as a cause of changes. (Dewey, 1938/1991, 30–31) (Quoted in Johnson, 2007, 10, our ellipses)

In other words, for SEA, there is no difference in kind but a continuous strand from the most basic organisms to humans. Mark Johnson (2007) goes on to explain, as he develops an embodied account of our cognitive capacities, that there is: (1) a higher-lower continuity whereby "higher" organisms are not unique evolutionarily, and where "higher" faculties (reason, will) are not different in kind from "lower" ones (emotion, perception) and (2) an inner-outer continuity whereby inner processes (mental) are not ontologically different from outer ones (physical) (122).

In short, rather than splits, SEA posits holistic continuities of actual processes and maintains connections among phenomena rather than divisions in "kind," extending from simple organisms to persons, from minimal to complex cognitive processes, and from nonrepresentational to scaffolded, enculturated cognition. As we will discuss in connection to Dewey's body-mind, this also eschews dualist accounts of mind and body (as well as brain and body, which implies dualism in the sense that the brain acts as the mind, see Bennett & Hacker, 2003). Importantly, this continuity does not imply lack of meaningful distinctions or boundaries within experience. Rather these differentiations arise "against the background of continuous processes" (Johnson, 2007, 122).

To return to Cox's 10-mile swim: the environment is comprised of those features that are "alive" and pertinent for Cox. These include the ocean and its relevant facets—currents (weak, strong), water (temperature, salinity, turbidity), waves (size, direction, speed)—meteorological conditions (approaching gales), time of day (nighttime or daylight), entourage (teammates or competitors if present, support crews), fauna (aggressive sharks, dolphins, whales—all of which she has encountered)—and her history of engagements (familiarity with waters and crews is peremptory for safe passages). As Bredo (1994) puts it, "it may help to think of a performance as the product of a history of relating, in which both person and environment change over the course of the transaction" (28). In contrast to CRS's static symbolic models, and very much following the tide of the SEA, Cox actively and dynamically adapts to the fluid waves, and the water itself "responds" differently to her varying stroke speeds, movement patterns, and techniques (entry and exit hand angles). She also adjusts her pace to fit unfolding conditions much as if she were dancing with the waves. Kinesthetic, kinetic, and tactile dynamics—how her body resonates directly to the aqueous environment—are central to this experience (Sheets-Johnstone, 2009).

These interactions become more nuanced with accumulated experience, prowess, fitness level, motivation, and deliberations before, during, and after performance. This is observable in Cox's own narrative. As she swims across the frigid waters of Alaska's Glacier Bay, amid small yet dangerous icebergs and sharp-edged sheets of ice, Cox (2014) writes,

> The intensity of this swim was like nothing I had ever experienced. It was unbelievable. There was so *much to be aware of*, and yet, throughout it all, I had to stay *absolutely focused* on how my body was responding. The icebergs I passed seemed to be exhaling breaths of icy air. Despite the cold, I was enjoying the swim. It was absolutely beautiful, seeing the icebergs dancing in the water currents, watching them as they changed colors—blue, green, white, silver, and gold—and brightened with light and deepened with shadow. (217, our emphases)

It is remarkable that while pushing herself in such perilous conditions, she is capable of being intensely focused (monitoring water currents, her course, support boat) and, more extraordinary yet, that she can also notice and enjoy the haze and iridescences in the icebergs she swims by. Crucially, this is connected to skilled performance.

Experienced sea and river people read water, rapids, and waves as easily as readers parse these words. When looking at turbulent rapids, most people on a whitewater rafting or kayaking trip see "chaos. But a good boatman [sees] order and opportunity" so that when one avenue deteriorates, others reveal themselves (Deurbrouck, 2012, 189). This is a matter of situated and cultivated skill. Jo Deurbrouck elaborates on whitewater experts: "That was the point of polishing your skills and honing your judgment. Skill and judgment transformed an uncontrollable environment into one of managed risk. Skill and judgment gave you the right to ride" (2012, 189). Much as consummate oenologists detect an impressive number of chemical compounds in wine unnoticeable to both neophytes and most who indulge in Bacchanalian pursuits, expert sportspeople develop their skills and are capable of lifting off intricate and refined experiential features from the complex phenomena that their extreme kinetic engagements afford them (Ilundáin-Agurruza, 2016).

The long interactions and exposures of ultra events offer the opportunity to explore in detail environmental and personal changes and adaptations at many different levels and in various states, from perceptions of sensorial stimuli to—as fatigue increases—variations along the full emotional arc (in relation to physical and psychic perceptions), and even how judgment is affected under duress. More importantly, the extended temporal dimension allows for personal transformation. Additionally, there are also rich and complex social and cultural aspects to this individual-environment coupling with different roles that range from the merely contextual to the constitutive (section five discusses personal transformation and the social dimension). Obviously, sportspersons need to be attentive and reflective enough to take advantage of such occasions, but *ceteris paribus* their skills and the situations they are able to handle open experiential spaces foreclosed to most others.

Vitally, this is a fully embodied process. Dewey refers to the "body-mind" in order to emphasize the continuity of psychophysical phenomena. Johnson (2007) explains,

> According to Dewey's principle of continuity, what we call "body" and "mind" are simply convenient abstractions—shorthand ways of identifying aspects of ongoing organism-environment interactions—so cognition, thought, and symbolic interaction . . . must be understood as arising from organic processes. (117)

Dewey closely followed the psychology, science, and research of what today would be called sciences of the mind (cognitive science, neuroscience, etc.). His naturalized view of minds sought alignment with empirical research. On the contemporary scene, defenders of radical forms of enactivism espouse key elements of Dewey's approach—an understanding of habits as world-directed and context-sensitive, placing habit at the heart of mind.

Enactivism denies that mental representations are the basis for cognition and skills. By its lights, cognition is a matter of relating and responding, not representing. Cognitive processes do not stand behind and cause intelligent behavior but rather they themselves unfold and take shape through an organism's active exploration of and engagement with aspects of the world (Hutto and Myin, 2013; 2017). Basic cognition exhibits intentionality, that is, organisms *target and are directed* at worldly situations. Such world-directed activity, however, is not intensional (with-an-s), which would entail the existence of *semantic* meanings or contents that have conditions of satisfaction. Subverting Fodor's famous mantra, according to the radically enactivist approach, there is no representation without interaction.[4]

Radical enactivists advance a complex view of cognition. They do not hold that all thinking is contentless. For them, content-involving thought—exemplified by propositional reasoning—is possible for some creatures. Yet it requires mastery of a special kind of intersubjective practice built atop and upon the exercise of contentless forms of cognition. Thus, radical enactivism seeks to understand both contentless basic forms of cognition and content-involving forms of cognition and how they interact. It supplies a two-tiered, multifaceted account of cognitive phenomena—such as imagination and memory—that CRS cognitivist rivals think as representational through and through (Hutto, 2015; Hutto and Myin, 2017). Recent work argues that radical enactivist accounts supply powerful resources for understanding the highly sophisticated cognition in action typical of sports and martial arts (Ilundáin-Agurruza, 2016, 2017b; Ilundáin-Agurruza, Krein & Erickson, 2018; Krein & Ilundáin Agurruza, 2017).[5]

Whitewater kayakers often use topographic maps and hydrographic data when planning a trip, thereby relying on external representations. Once amid the turbulent waters, however, even as they "read" the water, it is possible to understand such cognitive processes without assuming them to be rooted in contentful mental representations. Rather, the kayakers are immediately responsive and immersed in the thick of the action. Their skillful corporeal imaginings (Ilundáin-Agurruza, 2017a) open them to opportunities to perform foreclosed to those less experienced. Fully in the moment, they act based on their history of whitewater engagements. Their skilled kinetic repertoire affords different possible ways, some better than others, to explore what the world has to offer and to fluidly and dynamically adapt to such offerings. Once the kayakers dock, they can tell tall or short tales of their exploits and reflectively analyze their performance. *Then*, our "epistemic tendrils" interweave contentless and contentful states. But these, as well as our more refined practices for which semantic content is key, are hard won scaffolded achievements, not resources that are a feature of our basic minds.

On the SEA, the organism-environment coupling also affects our understanding of the boundaries of cognition. To embrace a radical enactive vision is to surrender the idea that cognition is not limited to brain, body, or person in favor of the view that it is extensive: it is integrated with and spans body-mind and environment, where the latter is inclusive of tools.[6] The social ramifications of this stance are examined in section five; for now suffice it to say that an extensive view of basic cognition envisions it as always, already world-involving. In this case, neither organism nor its environment is favored regarding our cognitive engagements. To remain with watercraft, consummately skilled boat people often identify with their rig—notably those who have built their boats, such as Joshua Slocum, who first sailed around the world alone, and for whom his boat was "a little bark which of all man's handiwork seemed to me nearest to perfection of beauty" (Slocum, 1956, 3). Dame Ellen MacArthur, (2005) who also circumnavigated the earth—albeit unassisted and continuously—speaks of her boat, *Kingfisher,* not as a tool or as even a mere extension of her, but rather as a symbiosis: they become one as they careen up and down the wild waves of the Southern Seas, making over twenty knots amid treacherous icebergs that could put a swift end to *them*. *Kingfisher* through its hull, mast, and rigging transmits to MacArthur the full register of oceanic and meteorological conditions so they become part of a transactional performance with the windy and wavy environment.

Significantly, the capacity for intense transaction with the environment is trainable. In other words, it can (and should) be actively fostered and habituated. How ultra athletes become more attuned to the environment and learn how to have stimulating dialogues with it takes us to the next waypoint and ratchets up the intensity.

## IN THE TOSS AND THICK OF THE ACTION: DEWEYAN HABIT AND DELIBERATION

Habit and deliberation are prominent in Dewey's work, and crucial to bringing the best out of us, whether it be in life or ultra events. They enable skill tempering and character polishing so that risks are faced squarely, and success or failure duly managed. In this section we examine each sequentially, noting upfront that these intimately intertwine when implemented, and that the segregated discussion is for conceptual clarity.

Dewey's conception of habit, a term he bemoaned and adopted for practicality, is anything but what the Oxford English Dictionary defines as, "A settled or regular tendency or practice, especially one that is hard to give up."

It is commonly thought also that developing a habit is a matter of mere repetition, and that achieving it singularly relies on will power driving the effort. Habit is also often associated with intellectual realization: if one understands the matter, then one can also forge a way.

Characteristically, Dewey turns this on its head. For him, habits are not static and repetitive "reflex-like" actions but rather dynamic processes. These processes act as conditions of intellectual efficiency that restrict the intellect (Dewey, 1988).[7] In doing so, they provide us with alternative ways of engaging the environment. Accordingly, habits are situated. In this way, they are catalysts of transformative processes and self-cultivating dispositions. Further, unlike blind mechanisms, Deweyan habits are flexible and context-sensitive (Gallagher & Miyahara, 2012; note that this aligns well with Merleau-Ponty's notion of habit, see Butler and Gallagher, 2018). Moreover, willing is not what enables habits. On the contrary, habits are needed to mediate between wishes and their implementation. Considering the example of good posture, Dewey says, those who *can* stand do so, and only a man who can does (Dewey, 1988).

To distinguish his view from the term's usual associations, and to emphasize the point that it is more fruitfully conceived as a skill, we adopt the coinage of "skilled habit" (SH) to identify Dewey's view. SHs act as limitations that we hone as we strive to improve. But, these constraints also open spaces to perform: "Habits become negative limits because they are first positive agencies" (Dewey, 1988, 123). In pruning inefficiencies, SH actually fosters creative spaces, for we need to improvise, adapt, and deliberate to meet challenges. When the challenges are as sobering as those ultraendurance sportspeople embrace, SH serves them better than a traditional approach to habit. If Dewey is being descriptive, the very concepts are concurrently prescriptive. After all, how we conceive of habits also influences how we implement them.

The subjacent ethos of ultraendurance seems to be constituted of endless repetitive acts. But, here the fallacy of composition—that something is true of the whole because it is true of a part of the whole—is given the lie by the exploits of ultra athletes. When famed mountaineer and adventurer Reihhold Messner, the first person to climb Everest without supplemental oxygen, took ten million steps (give or take a couple) to cross Antarctica on foot, it was not simply the mere addition of a discrete number of steps. Rather, the exploit was the aggregation of the full experience where the steps coalesced into qualitative assemblages that constitute an adventure (we discuss Dewey's notion of experience below). A traditional view of habit reinforces the repetitive and molds an ensconced, predictable existence whereas SH allows us to thrive as we explore transactionally an ever broadening, deepening environment.

Consider next that for Dewey (1922), "a habit is a form of executive skill, of *efficiency in doing*" (55, our emphasis). This efficiency is concretely body-minded in the economy of movement that expert ultra athletes develop, as the smallest inefficiencies are magnified exponentially over such extended performances. What may cost but a handful of seconds over a flat kilometer will add up to hours over uneven terrain as fatigue accentuates unskilled inefficiencies. To tie this to a previous central idea, these performances are not simply a matter of athletic talent and determination but, in a truly situated fashion, they pertain to the environment as much as to the individual: "We are perhaps apt to emphasize the control of the body at the expense of control of the environment" (Dewey, 1922, 55). Running, skiing, sailing, climbing, swimming, are usually, and rightly, thought of as specialized skills for athletes, a matter of prowess and precision. "They are that, of course," Dewey agrees as he goes on to clarify, "but the measure of the value of these qualities lies in the economical and effective control of the environment which they secure" (ibid.). Executing this "is to have certain properties of nature at our disposal" (ibid.).

Offshore sailing illustrates this well, specifically the ultimate challenge: The Vendée Globe Regatta. Sailors circumnavigate the globe alone without stops or assistance. Finishers take from two and a half to five months; those less fortunate sail off to never return. Sailors worth their salt are keenly aware that it is the environment that hones their SHs. Different waters and winds, and their many moods, need different skills and habits, for example, the treacherous waters off Cape Horn, or the maddening windless days where the directionless cork-like bobbing elicits existential ennui. In 2005, Ellen MacArthur broke the world record for fastest solo circumnavigation, setting it at 71 days, 14 hours, and a handful of minutes. MacArthur's sailing talent is best accounted for in terms of SH, for this allows her to be "intellectually at home on the sea," as Dewey (1988) opportunely phrases matters (121).

Navigating troubled waters—sailing, in life—requires, besides skills and dynamically responsive habits, skilled deliberation. Situated interactions are ideally harmonious but realistically discordant. Oftentimes, because of the multiplicity of perspectives and interests, these transactions lead to conflict. Then, Bredo (1994) explains, "their resolution depends on finding a way of approaching the situation that successfully defines it in a way that makes it solvable, allowing the activity to proceed" (24). The way to solve some conflicts, however, is not through a *narrow* interpretation of Aristotelian deliberation as linear, however successful it may be in many contexts.

A linear Aristotelian model of deliberation, James Wallace (2009) explains, when intended to cover all cases of deliberations, "implies that we are equipped at the outset with clearly and concretely articulated purposes, goals, or ends that will provide us with our starting point of deliberation"

(22). In some cases, there is a clear predicament for which the sought outcome is plainly defined: a torn sail needs to be mended, and the solution is patching and sewing, or replacement by another sail if available. Then, the linear account is unquestionably suitable. Yet, there are other "challenging practical circumstances [for which], however, we are not guided at the outset by a concrete conception of the outcome we want" (Wallace, 2002, 22). Some incommensurate and conflicted situations have no clear answer. Wallace points out that we want to be fair to all, "But what is that in *this* particular situation?" (ibid., 22–23, our emphasis). The *strictly* linear approach is problematically inflexible.

Dewey broadens the interpretation, building on Aristotelian *phronesis*—a skillful and sound practical judgment. He develops an imaginative *phronesis* (IP) that is dynamic and creative. For Dewey (1988), the way forward is by means of "a dramatic rehearsal (in imagination) of various competing possible lines of action" that arrests express action and curbs established habits (132). A salient point is that for Dewey deliberation is not a matter of algorithmic elimination of possibilities or mere heuristic shortcuts. Instead, it is subject to a process of nurtured SH: "To be able to single out a definitive sensory element in any field is evidence of a high degree of previous training, that is, of well-formed habits" (Dewey, 1988, 25). This involves "a search for *a way* to act, not for a final terminus" (ibid., 134, Dewey's emphasis). The true import of this insight comes forth in the next section when we consider ends and means.

Sporting competitive contexts "complicate" the simple structure that constitutes games—achieving a goal through inefficient means. Hence, what seems to be a paradigmatic case for Aristotelian deliberation is best seen in (terms of) IP. The success/failure (win/loss) dyad easily leads to multiple ways of going about achieving the primary goal. It is not simply about aiming to succeed (or win), but of *how* to go about it. There are multiple ways to succeed or fail. One can break rules or honor them variously, from creative cheating to questionable adherence to rules, for example, taking products or using technologies that are legal and performance enhancing but against the spirit of the rules: hypoxic chambers (Clarey N.D.), the to-this-day WADA legal[8] sodium phosphate that Joel Friel (2003) recommends in his *Cyclist's Training Bible* (pp. 220–221), Nike's controversial secret running program (Hart, 2017). Or, one can supererogatorily go beyond the rules, as when helping competitors even against one's self-interest. Italian bobsledder Eugenio Monti is superlatively inspiring: he loaned a vital piece to the British team that won the Olympic gold over the Italians. Sailors and mountaineers sometimes need to choose between a goal they may have prepared for a lifetime or helping someone in straits (perhaps due to negligence). What if this person is a sibling, or a daughter? What if trying to help risks the safety of the whole group? Fair play in sport is also a complex issue, as competitors ought to win fairly but, for some, this does not entail that fair play as abiding by the rules is tantamount to moral duty (Bysted Moller and Moller, 2015).

Deliberation can take on a rather sharp yet still incommensurate character, as Cox's (2014) ruminations illustrate:

> Thirty-two degrees. That was a magic number, the temperature at which freshwater froze. I wondered if in thirty-two-degree water the water in my cells would freeze, if my body's tissues would become permanently damaged. I wondered if my mind would function better this time, if I would be able to be more aware of what was happening, or if it would be further dulled by the cold. Would my core temperature drop faster, more quickly than I could recognize? Would I be able to tell if I needed to get out? Did I really want to risk my life for this? Or did I want to risk failure? The other part of me wanted to try, wanted to do what I had trained for, wanted to explore and reach beyond what I had done. (345)

For her, there is no easy way to decide. As she avows, this "swim to Antarctica was the culmination of thirty years of swimming and two years of complete focus on one big goal" (Cox, 2014, 358).

The Deweyan combination of skilled habit (SH) and imaginative *phronesis* (IP), combined into (SHIP), provides a perspective that permits navigating through rough situations and finding *a* way. SHIP provides a subtle, situated, context-sensitive ability for tacking and maneuvering, as opposed to the mere application of utilitarian calculation or deontological rule application. Aristotelian *phronesis* is then integrated into a dynamic model that is *particularized* to the needs of the specific situation and whose solution is arrived at much as a doctor draws a diagnosis. The point is that "the good achieved is unique to the situation and is discovered and articulated *only* as a result of deliberations" (Wallace, 2009, 23 his emphasis). The solution is not preset but, much as in athletic abilities, it is skillfully found in the doing. A flexible approach to deliberation is all the more pertinent, from a situated stance, because "our environment changes continually, and we must constantly adapt our practices to unforeseen developments" (ibid., 25). It may not necessarily lead to a happy result. Some heart-wrenching decisions, such as those illustrated by sailing and mountaineering above, just exclude such possibility. Still, SHIP is more capable of discriminating in a fine textured way, and this offers not only better guidance, but also a modicum of solace in reassuring us that we *did* consider *all* sensible angles.

As a whole, the SEA requires a radically situated and enactive process that hinges on active, dynamically habituated body-minds. By training our body-mind we can perform better. In doing so, our body-mind is not a mere means. Or, rather, it *is* a means indeed but no mere instrument. This has momentous import for how we come to understand and practice ultraendurance sports.

## WHEN THE GOING GETS TOUGH: ENDS AS MEANS AND RISKY LESSONS

Ever original and dynamic, Dewey also redefines the relation between means and ends, connecting it to habit.[9] Together with radical enactivism, the hypothesis is that this brings transparency to the "inner" workings of the type of skilled performance unique to these sports. Further, it can also refine our understanding of and provide a better model on which to base an appreciation for the process of ultraendurance sport activity where the goal of meaningful completion is not merely end-oriented. In this way it is also aligned with, or rather, builds on SHIP, for as Dewey (1922) states, "A habit means an ability to use natural conditions as means to ends" (55). We explore the radical implications of this stance next.

Kilian Jornet Burgada is a 29-year-old ultra skyrunner (running up and down mountains) whose record-breaking is record-setting itself. Denali takes experienced climbers up to two weeks to summit. Jornet run it in 9 hours and 43 minutes. In 2017, as part of his "Summits of My Life Project," he summited Mount Everest in record time from 11,000 ft Everest Base Camp to the top's 29,000 ft in 26 hours. From a higher camp, he summited again two days later barely missing another record. Such exploits, impressive as they may be, are like any other goal seeking action. The inner structure of intentional action concerns means and ends, and our valuation of these. But, the conventional account of instrumental rationality offers a questionable analysis of instrumentality and intrinsic/extrinsic value in relation to means and ends. Basically, it is a dualistic stance that clearly and distinctly distinguishes means from ends. Instrumental rationality also advances the idea that the value of the means is found extrinsically, as these are taken as instruments to other goods or objectives, whereas ends are viewed as noninstrumental and thus intrinsically valuable. Money, then, is a means of solely extrinsic value, happiness an intrinsically valuable end, and health a hybrid of sorts.

In this classification, sports are instrumentally used whenever health, wealth, or fame is *exclusively* sought. But, as Mike McNamee (2008) observes, sports are non-utilitarian if highly instrumental in that they are gratuitous difficulties that we invent. That is, designed as artificial challenges, sports are but superfluous endeavors. This does not entail that sports can only be engaged instrumentally. Yet, some make an instrument of instrumental rationality itself to suit their own purposes so that the ends justify the means. This often leads to competition as a zero-sum endeavor where wins are achieved at the expense of those losing, and all too often results in unsporting behavior (e.g., cheating, doping). It also endorses results over processes: what matters is the podium place or record, rather than the experience. Given the paltriness or even absence of monetary rewards in many ultra events athletes often fashion themselves as a counterculture inured to such "warped" tendencies. Besides, record-breaking in these sports remains a rather anonymous affair that circumvents stardom (it is a safe bet that many readers will not recognize most ultra athletes mentioned in this chapter). Nonetheless, yet predictably, there are cheaters and dopers among "ultras" (Brown, 2016). Tackling these morally suspect sporting practices is beyond the scope of this chapter, but a situated approach changes the terms of engagement so that the passion for the activity itself comes first thereby making such questionable actions if not irrelevant at least unappealing.

Garrett Thomson (2003) argues that instrumental rationality is mistaken: it assumes the instrumentality of means and the noninstrumentality of ends. Accordingly, when action is concerned, goals alone are noninstrumental. But, this denies the action itself of having any value because if something is valuable as an instrument to something or for someone else then it is not valuable in itself. In other words, if something is purely instrumental—as the standard view posits—then that implies that it is not valuable itself as its worth lies solely in how it is useful to the goal. On the contrary, Thomson (2003) argues, we should never treat our "actions merely instrumentally" (51). We can argue that people, activities, and actions themselves are meaningful (and valuable) insofar as we engage them noninstrumentally. "It is a matter of how we should conceive the good: the good should not be defined as an aim" (Thomson, 2003, 52). Without trivializing ends or results, this allows for the process to gain in significance. Critically, it does not do so at the cost of emphasizing process over results or means over ends.

As mentioned, an instrumentally narrow rational approach makes competition the point of the activity, and within it, winning the contest becomes the primary objective. Serious athletes, definitely those of Jornet's caliber, orient their training accordingly: schedules alternate light and heavy workloads and intensity, which are methodically organized around key competitions; "techno-gadgets" that correlate GPS tracked routes to wattage output, calories, heart rate, and other metrics are used extensively; calories are fastidiously counted. This makes for precise goals and rational training plans that seek maximum return on investment: a better shot at winning.

Jornet begs to differ. He races almost weekly, something unheard of at the elite level, and instead of gizmos, training plans, and special diets, Jornet just gets lost in the mountains for seven or eight hours a day, often stopping to talk to locals and hikers (McDougal 2014). Distinctively, even if Jornet *does* try to win races, he views them lightheartedly. As Jornet puts it, "This sport is about improving, not winning" and suggests, "You never learn from victory" (McDougall, 2014, 73). As expected, the proof is in the plodding: in his first Western States, a famed U.S. ultra race, he was battling it out for the lead when he leaped and clicked his heels à la Fred Astaire, because, "you have to *make* some fun. What we do isn't serious" (ibid., our emphasis).

Jornet incarnates a different understanding of his sporting trade that belies traditional views and the competitive ethos that instrumental rationality underwrites. For Jornet training *and* competing are not different: it is all about the running experience, or rather, the experiences that skyrunning affords in the mountains. As fellow competitor Dakota Jones (one of a few to have beat Jornet) explained: "The week before Hardrock [where he beat Jornet], he ran like five hours on the course every day. Crazy! But he'd never been there before and wanted to check out the scenery" (McDougall, 2014, 73) In Jornet's words: "Such beautiful mountains! I went out, met people, ran the summits, the rivers. It's a shame if you just go there to race" (ibid.).

This aligns neatly with the present situated stance. Dewey (1988) asserts, "Means and ends are two names for the same reality" (27). Differently put, the ends become instrumental for the means and become one and the same; it is only perspective that marks the difference. Dewey explains, "Means are means; they are intermediates, middle terms. *To grasp this fact is to have done with the ordinary dualism of means and ends.* The 'end' is merely a series of acts viewed at a remote stage; and a means is merely the series viewed at an earlier one" (1988, 26, our emphasis). Concordantly, the means already contain the end. In this case, if the means do not contain/reflect the character of the end, then they will transform the nature of the end itself, for example, fostering democratic athletes does not result from autocratic coaches.[10] In short, the distinction is not ontological but rather relational and context-dependent. This shines the spotlight on the activity itself while reinvesting ends into the loop. In short, goals and ends give us reason(s) to do what we enjoy.

In this model, ends are instrumentally valuable because they further activity. Thomson (2003) puts it memorably, "The ends are means to the means" (52). More prosaically, he clarifies, "goals are means to non-instrumentally valuable activities, which are also means" (ibid.). Moreover, objectives "are not intrinsically valuable even if they direct and explain action" (ibid., 53). We may have the goal of building a surfboard, yet surfboards are but part of larger processes that make for more wave-riding. Thus, even if the surfboard was the goal, it was so but instrumentally. As Thomson explains, this confusion arises because "it is the goals of our activities that are instrumentally valuable; they are valuable to achieve because they lead to further worthwhile activities" (ibid.). For those who, like Jornet, embrace training and competition thusly, crossing finish lines or reaching summits is but a way to more running or climbing—the kind that leads to improving and learning.

This ethos leads to fulsome experiences: those that are vital and to which "we spontaneously refer to as being 'real experiences,'" and about which "we say in recalling them, 'that *was* an experience'" (Dewey, 1980, 36). Sometimes these are memorably poignant and intense. In 2012, Jornet attempted to set the record for speed crossing of the Mont Blanc massif, running alongside sky/mountaineer Stéphane Brosse. He writes, "An instant is what separates happiness from pain. Everything is decided in millimeters, in tenths of a second. The cornice atop which Stéphane is breaks, taking him along with a great amount of snow" (Jornet, 2012, our translation). Brosse fell over 2,000 feet and died on impact. It could well have been Jornet, as he was on the inside and Brosse on the outside of the same cornice. After memorializing Brosse in a video where he discussed his philosophy on life (Ara, 2012), Jornet paid the most emotive and fitting tribute a year later: he broke the Mont Blanc record to honor Brosse.

The quality of such happenings is that of an experiential totality or a consummation, as it is "a whole and carries with it its own individualizing quality and self-sufficiency" (Dewey, 1980, 35). As such, this kind of experience is not discrete and atomistic but continuous in body-minded thought, perception, and feeling (Johnson, 2008, 122). Thus, it is the foundation of what Dewey called a "situation": "the whole complex of physical, biological, social, and cultural conditions that constitute any given experience" (ibid., 72). This, Dewey highlights as *an* experience that changes us inside out, and which he illustrates thus:

> Then, there is that storm one went through in crossing the Atlantic—a storm that seemed in its fury, as it was experienced, to sum up in itself all that a storm can be, complete in itself, standing out because marked out from what went before and what came after. (1980, 36)

Noteworthy experiences have the sense of an adventure where what is about to happen hangs on the line, a line demarcating the before and after.[11]

Ultraendurance sports are designed to foster such experiences. Since they are refined celebrations of pain, Dewey's observation that significant experience has "an element of suffering, in its large sense" because "otherwise there would be no taking in of what preceded" (ibid., 41), takes on added significance. This is especially true in sports and enterprises where prolonged effort is coupled to *genuine* risk.

Risk is inherent to ultraendurance events. They may include the risk of serious harm or death or be safer but still involve daunting challenges that may end in failure after much struggle. The underlying ethos involves finding our limits and then pushing against them. Sensibly Cox (2005) states that no record is worth one's life, but that does not mean that life is valuable to the point of excluding all risk. Risk may be a source of self-affirmation, as John Russell (2006) argues regarding risk sports. Moreover, as Messner (2014) avows, engaging risk is a matter of safety not security. Concurring with Jornet, Messner sees that the value of formidable trials is not found in success; rather failure is a more powerful experience because it is where we truly find our limits. Further, when "you fail the objective remains" (Messner, 2014, 116). Despair may follow, but this can be a stimulus "to understand the failure, [and] comprehend your own limits" (ibid.). Appositely for a situated stance where skills are central, Messner says that "to fail well requires practice" (2014, 116). When Ricardo Abad set as his challenge fifty Ironman in as many consecutive days, then quit after only three days, he was completely "crushed and feeling absolutely awful" (Marca, 2014, our translation). After so many unbelievable records, Abad was not ready to fail, much less so early into his challenge.

Taking on veritable risks where we may spectacularly fail can help us grow. Trepidation and fear are to be expected when we put ourselves to the test and, in certain scenarios, they are the price tag for new experiences. When speaking about his respect and fear of the mountain and how he seeks safety, Jornet states that "we seek precisely that, to find new things (experiences), but that is also what we find fearful" (Piedrabuena, 2012a, our translation). Intimidated by the stakes, the initial reaction may be to shun such endeavors. This is problematic, as it drains our life of vitality. Hochstetler and Hopsicker (2012) write, "to avoid challenging opportunities leads to a life of stasis rather than growth" (124). On the one side, a life devoid of such personal adventures becomes existentially parochial and limiting. On the other side, excessive adventuring and overly strenuous pursuits without reflection lead to existential opacity.

The darker side of ultraendurance culture lies in overexertion, which imprudently overplays late whitewater guide Clancy Reece's dictum, "anything worth doing is worth overdoing" (Deurbrouck, 2012). Murakami (2008) reflects a similar sentiment: "If something's worth doing, it's worth giving it your best—or in some cases beyond your best" (89). Discipline and persistence are the hammer and anvil that forge the ultra indomitability, but often they result in inflexibility, uncreative doggedness, and stultifying habits. This frequently leads to injuries and burnout. It should be clear that a Deweyan flexible habit and dynamic deliberation is able to temper matters to bring the necessary suppleness to our character.

Fully experiencing process and results as equal opportunity partners and, besides enjoying successes, learning from our failures, all benefit from the sort of skilled practice that body-minded SHIPs nurture. A situated Deweyan approach to ultraendurance equips sportspersons not just with the tools to court success (talent, training, and luck have much to say), but also with the means to come out ahead, should worthy lessons be drawn, even in failure. Therein we find the fertile soil on which to thrive.

## FLOURISHING WITH THE SECOND WIND: PERSONAL DISCOVERY AND SOCIAL COGNITION

Ultra events are a modern version of the olden times explorers' *Terra Incognita*: the mystery that lay beyond the known world. Haruki Murakami's (2008) memoir on his lifelong pursuit of running guides us in this uncharted region. Discoursing on his 62-mile ultramarathon around Lake Saroma in Hokkaidō (Japan), he writes:

> For me this was the Strait of Gibraltar, beyond which lay an unknown sea. What lay in wait beyond this, what unknown creatures were living there, I didn't have a clue. In my own small way I felt the same fear that sailors of old must have felt. (Murakami, 106)

The race was very meaningful for him as a runner even if the "general significance of running sixty-two miles by yourself" was unclear to him (Murakami, 2008, 104). But, since running that long is not an ordinary event, "you'd expect it to afford you a special sort of self-awareness. It should add a few new elements to your inventory in understanding who you are" (ibid.). Precisely, ultraendurance gifts us with opportunities for self-understanding and transformation. Murakami continues, "as a result, your view of your life, its colors and shape, should be transformed. More or less, for better or for worse, this happened to me, and I was transformed" (ibid.). These transformations, like the metamorphosis from chrysalis to butterfly or moth, are neither always easy nor do they always result in beauty. Murakami lost his zeal for running: "I ended up with was a sense of lethargy . . . I felt covered by a thin film, something I've since dubbed runner's blues. (Though the actual feeling of it was closer to a milky white)" (Murakami, 2008, 116). He lost his enthusiasm for the act of running itself. It would be a long time before he felt a renewed natural desire "to get out on the road and run, just like when I'm dehydrated and crave the juice from a fresh piece of fruit" (Murakami, 2008, 120).

Yet, Murakami (2008) affirms that "Even now I'm glad I ran the race" in spite of having "to deal with these aftereffects somehow" (118). Why he *still* embraces the race, we can surmise, is partially due to a new kind of experience. All he could think near the finish of a marathon was to end it, but as he completed the ultramarathon,

> I wasn't really thinking about this. The end of the race is just a temporary marker without much significance. It's the same with our lives. . . . An end point is simply set up as a temporary marker, or perhaps as an indirect metaphor for the fleeting nature of existence. It's very philosophical—not that at this point

I'm thinking how philosophical it is. I just vaguely experience this idea, not with words, but as a physical sensation. (Murakami, 2008, 114–115)

This corresponds with how a situated body-mind operates during extreme performance. There is no propositional thinking that would count as contentful states, but just the action itself as the organism creates a joint kinetic expression with the environment and their transactional history. Murakami (2008) sheds light, explaining that once his fatigue vanished after the forty-seventh mile, "my mind went into a blank state you might even call philosophical or religious. Something urged me to become more introspective, and this newfound introspection transformed my attitude toward the act of running" (116–117). Paradoxically, this look within oneself eradicates the ego.

This disappearance of the self through strenuous effort has a long history in Japan's *dō* (道, Paths or ways of practice), which nurture growth through mindful movement. The practice of *iaidō* (居合道), the way of drawing out the sword, would count as ultraendurance nowadays in some cases. Hayashizaki Temple's records show that the top three swordsmen performed over 90,000 draws over a seven-day period—over 13,000 times a day (Tokitsu, 2004, 290). Within Buddhist soteriology the very pain and intense effort sought to overcome personal limitations, cultivate skillful fluency, and silence obvert contentful thinking. This gradually eliminates the self to an emptiness that Murakami (2008) also seeks: "really as I run, I don't think much of anything worth mentioning. I just run. I run in a void. Or maybe I should put it the other way: I run in order to acquire a void" (16). This process may result in a state of focused and mindfully fluid awareness called *mushin* (無心) in Japan (in the West "flow" designates a similar state, but without underlying Buddhist/Japanese cultural undertones).[12]

It is difficult to achieve and maintain such empty states. Lally (2013) explains, quoting Murphy, this creates,

> moments of present choice [that] are significant for just this reason: they make the world other than it is . . . This moral choice is an effective agent in the world, and it is this fact which gives meaning and zest to life. Indeed, this is Dewey's call to the heroic life. (193)

Ultraendurance creates experiences where pain, as a full body-minded phenomenon, demarcates a before and an after. Pain is necessary, Murakami (2008) explains, because:

> If pain weren't involved, who in the world would ever go to the trouble of taking part in sports like the triathlon or the marathon, which demand such an investment of time and energy? *It's precisely because of the pain, precisely because*

*we want to overcome that pain, that we can get the feeling, through this process, of really being alive*—or at least a partial sense of it. (170, our emphasis)

Worthy epiphanies must be paid for in comparable vital resources. In the case of ultraendurance, it is the expenditure of our limited energy in superfluous endeavors that is sacrificially offered in exchange for Sophia's wise revelations. Such epistemic transaction is not a *one-time* special occasion but rather a matter of relentless dedication and focus built on an uncompromising lifestyle fully dedicated to the "trade." The serious athlete preparing for a triathlon, Lally (2013) recounts, centers her life on the varied and daily workouts in swimming, cycling and running, nutrition, and rest, as "it is through these habits that we can come to know her" (179). These habits build the organism-environment transactional history of expert sportspersons.

Dewey advocated self-cultivation to our fullest potential while rejecting specific instructions that would lead us by the hand, Lally (2013) explains. In this context, the Japanese tradition of *shugyō* (修行), premised on lifelong practice in pursuit of flourishing and perfection, is expedient.[13] Translating and adequately rendering its Japanese connotations is difficult, but conceptually and practically, *shugyō* is closer to the underlying implications of Dewey's situated views than the usual notion of "self-cultivation." Cultivation is related to a tilling of the land, and the ideas of refinement and education. Yet, as Yuasa Yasuo (1993) points out, "the Japanese word . . . carries the sense of strengthening the mind (spirit) and enhancing the personality, as a human being, by training the body" (10). Significantly, the original Japanese words for "body" and "mind" (spirit)—*shintai* (身体) and *seishin* (精神), respectively—are phenomenologically endowed with rich "body-minded" associations (Ilundáin-Agurruza, 2016, Ch. 9). *Shugyō*, viewed as never ending because perfection is clearly unattainable, is a personal flourishing that is not tantamount to mere intellectual revelation; rather, it is truly *incarnate* in the fully body-minded practices of Japanese *dō*.

Presently then, we render *shugyō* as a resilient and enduring skillful striving (Ilundáin-Agurruza, 2016), as this captures the process of skilled adaptation through which organisms endeavor to flourish as they confront environmental challenges. In this fashion, it is readily and directly applicable to ultra practices. Murakami (2008) helps articulate this:

Running day after day, piling up the races, bit by bit I raise the bar, and by clearing each level I elevate myself. At least that's why I've put in the effort day after day: to raise my own level. I'm no great runner . . . But that's not the point. The point is whether or not I improved over yesterday. In long-distance running the only opponent you have to beat is yourself, the way you used to be. (10)

This is broadly applicable to ultraendurance sports. Nonetheless, there is an important difference. Whereas in Japan *dō* involve *explicit* self-reflection, and this attitude percolates other practices and Japanese culture generally, this is missing as such in the West (Carter, 2008). Ultra sportspeople could benefit from overt reflective habits; their experiences could become more significant in Dewey's sense, then. The following illustrates one of Murakami's (2008) running insights, "Your *quality of experience is based* not on standards such as time or ranking, but on finally *awakening to an awareness of the fluidity within action itself*" (170, our emphases). This is perfectly in sync with the views endorsed so far, centered on mindful awareness, movement, ends as means, and skillful fluidity.

Nevertheless, this is Murakami's *personal* realization. Just as pain is an individual's own, such epistemic revelations are intimate, nontransferable, and must be *lived* through rather than being contemplated as intellectual "lessons." Reading about others' insights may be inspiring, but just as studying all the manuals on sailing or climbing does not lead to *actual* know-how, this will not make us participate in *their* intimate truths. Regardless, this does not mean that we come into such epiphanies alone. Of course, personal discoveries can be expressed and communicated, and for those who partake of the practice (or similar ones) these can disclose fresh perspectives. In this way, rich personal experiences and their significance arise in community.

For Dewey's situated model, and for the SEA, there is a "practical inseparability of individual task performance from social relationships" (Bredo, 1994, 31). Dewey exactingly and extensively connected his views on reality, body-mind, and education to social institutions and processes, particularly in relation to democracy. In his in-depth examination of self-cultivation via Dewey and James, Lally (2013) accentuates that this process is not a purely individual matter but rather needs a community, and indicates, concerning endurance athletes who embody such processes of self-discovery, that: "What is necessary is the profound feeling that such efforts improve the person, connecting the athlete to a world larger than himself, one that is rich in meaning" (180). In sum, the distillation of personal character happens through a communal still.

Alasdair MacIntyre (1984) has argued for and analyzed the role of communities, centered on practices, as the source of virtues of character, standards of excellence, and norms of conduct. McNamee (2008) has critically examined this stance in the context of sports as morality plays. From a situated perspective, the community has often been seen as instrumental in making these distillations personally and existentially relevant. But a stronger argument for the role of the community can be made: one where the community not only facilitates but also *constitutes* cognitive experiences typical of and central to specific practices. A practice can be portraiture painting in medieval times, as it is for MacIntyre (1994, 195), as much as ultrarunning in the twenty-first century. This furthers the previous discussion on extensive cognition.

A community built around a practice can play more than a merely supportive role in how it "organizes" cognitive experience. In a situated model cultural, institutional, and other environmental factors can be constitutive of and not simply contributing factors to the cognitive experience. Indeed, this experience is built up from the organism-environment transaction. A good case to consider before applying this model to ultraendurance sports is a "mental institution" without which the specific type of cognitive processes would not exist, for example, the legal system (Gallagher, 2013). Our cognitive processes are altered and extended to the degree that we engage legal "tools": legal institutions, contracts, and the justice system. Property rights, for instance, are too complex to keep it all "in mind." Convoluted cases cannot be limited to the brain; they benefit from a cognition that is distributed across different agents and levels. Successful operation depends on extraneural practices beyond the heads/brains of lawyers, jurists, judges, juries, etc. Thus, these practices "beyond the brain" allow working with and managing complicated, copious information. This makes possible judgments that would not happen otherwise. Accordingly, instead of a CRS model reliant on brain-bound semantic content we can think of cognitive engagements as in the SEA—as dynamic processes that rectify problems and modulate behavior and action in an interactive and transformative relation with the environment. In this case not only tools, techniques, or technologies, but also institutions, practices, and communities extend our cognitive span.

Framing this from the perspective of social cognition, which empirical studies show is not reducible to the operations of individual cognitive mechanisms, shows that this broader milieu impacts cognitive experiences across the explanatory board, encompassing all three: contextual factors, enabling conditions, and constitutive elements (De Jaegher, Di Paolo & Gallagher, 2010).[14] The constitutive elements, importantly, give us the qualitative uniqueness of the interactive experience; they make it what it is. The contextual and enabling conditions affect and scaffold interactions, but experiments show that in certain contexts, when agents are in a situation in which they can respond to their collective dynamics, "the interaction process is not only enabling but plays a constitutive role" (ibid., 445).

For us, just as the legal system exemplifies an extensive and socially situated cognition, ultraendurance practices, institutions, and communities parallel this. We find traditions, techniques, technologies, and ongoing kinetic judgments and actionable commitments that scaffold, distribute, and extend shared knowledge and the development of skills. In the case of sports and ultra events, the framework of a community of practitioners with a rich history provides many possibilities for interactive dynamics whereby participants respond to one another and learn skills that directly affect the quality and kind of their cognitive experiences. They sharpen their discriminatory powers to read water as sailors, SUP paddlers, and kayakers, or read rock, ice, snow, and winds as skiers and mountaineers. As they improve, they give back in kind. The central idea is that there is an *aggregation* of their skillful and experiential history with that of the community.

If Newton, by his own cognizance, stood on the shoulders of giants, here communities are the behemoths on which great feats are accomplished. Standouts like Cox and Jornet began precociously—Jornet summited his first 14,000-foot peak, the Breithorn, when he was 6 (Dumons, 2013); Cox swam the 27 miles from Catalina Island to the California coast at 14—the youngest to ever do that. If they could begin so early and go so far, it is because they unerringly benefited from strong communities that afforded requisite means and, above all, people. Cox trained alongside future Olympic champions and started under the tutelage of U.S. Olympic coach Don Gambril (Cox, 2014); Jornet progressed under the wing of the *Centre de Tecnificació d'Esquí de Muntanya de Catalunya* (CTEMC), which forms young people in the various modalities of mountain climbing, and about which Jornet avers, "when we begin to do sports, we need guides, people who love the sport and transmit that love and their knowledge" (Piedrabuena, 2012b, our translation). None of their records would have been possible without a nurturing and extensive entourage of people, whom both Cox and Jornet often gratefully credit. They take risks alongside them that could also imperil their lives: Brosse fell to his death during Jornet's first of his Summits of my Life project; others risked their boats or themselves in some of Cox' swims.

In sum, the exploits of phenomenal performers, however they may be lionized, are not only constituted by the means communities provide. Their innovations and feats become interwoven as one more aggregate to the tradition's communal tapestry. Cox showed that, with adaptation and requisite training, it was possible to swim and survive in Antarctic waters, for example. Others have taken up the challenge since, swimming in freezing waters around the world. Yet, this is not only or foremost about the stars of the sport; most are neither as talented, able, accomplished, or lucky. Some are latecomers: Murakami began running when he was 33. But in his own dedicated way—Murakami has run at least a marathon every year, often several—like countless others, he and they support their practices and communities in virtue of their modest contributions. They are the ones keeping the practices alive; they are the unsung heroes who anonymously constitute the giants on which legends stand.

## THE FINISH LINE: CONCLUDING REMARKS

In this chapter we have discussed the mutually beneficial relationship between ultraendurance endeavors and a Deweyan situated perspective. The former benefits greatly from a Deweyan inspired ethos while the latter finds an ideal and complicit partner for its implementation. A situated and enactive approach (SEA) to cognition highlights the transactional and organic coupling of organism/sportsperson and environment in ways that better describe the inner workings of such a finely tuned "performing ecosystem," and the highly developed sensorial discriminatory capacities that result in complexly rich cognitive experiences. An enactive model of cognition does away with burdensome mental representations and highlights the immediate and direct immersion of sportspersons. The body-mind, acting as a holistic unity that underscores the continuity among phenomena then flourishes through SHIP: a combined Deweyan skilled habit (SH) and reflectively adopted imaginative *phronesis* (IP) that constitutes a dynamic deliberation that complements the Aristotelian view. This SHIP sails on when facing head-on incommensurate alternatives that require discovery or redefinition of goals and means. Vital for this is a new way of looking at ends as means to the means such that we can be guided by objectives that emphasize the very activity itself. The momentous experiences that ultra sports make available profit from a situated approach, as it offers sensitive and sensible ways to engage and interpret them. This proves to be the best formula to help ultra practitioners flourish. It stimulates lifelong pursuits that arise within the enriching context of communitarian practices.

Ultra sports are anything but mindless, repetitive and monotonous pursuits where the finish line is all that matters, as conventional views paint them. As with any sport or game, they are superfluous undertakings. But, within a Deweyan framework, they arise as wholesome engagements in a life of kinetic inquiry and Socratic self-examination. Cox, Jornet, MacArthur, Messner, Murakami, and others give expression to and embody an ultraendurance kind of personal wisdom, inspiring us to follow them at our own pace. Dewey would approvingly nod and tie his shoelaces if given the chance.

## NOTES

1. This work was supported by the Australian Research Council Discovery Project "Minds in Skilled Performance" (DP170102987).
2. https://ultrasignup.com/register.aspx?did=42649 Accessed May 25, 2017.
3. Dewey favored "transaction" to avoid the dualistic connotations of "interaction."
4. Jerry Fodor writes that "there is No Intentional Causation without Explicit Representation" (1987, 25). In other words, for him there is "no computation without representation."

5. The competing CRS assumption that cognition is everywhere based on contentful mental representations that mediate between the world and us is philosophically problematic on a number of counts. Given the complexity of the arguments involved, it is sufficient to note that, due to the lack of a naturalistic theory of content, serious questions arise regarding the explanatory power that contentful mental representations can play, the lack of explanatorily robust means of assigning mental contents, and the want for an account of how contentful properties of mental representation make a causal difference in initiating and guiding intelligent behavior. These cast serious doubt on the familiar cognitivist idea that cognition necessarily involves content. For the radical enactive alternative, the intentionality and phenomenality of organisms' responses is not rooted in some type of knowledge but rather arises from concrete engagements or transactions with the environment. In basic acts of cognition, "there is not a set of facts that organisms know, or need to know, at any level" (Hutto and Myin, 2013, 30).

6. For a detailed argument for extensive minds in lieu of brain-bound or extended minds, see Hutto and Myin (2013, Ch. 8).

7. Intellect for Dewey, as the discussion of the body-mind should make clear, is an embodied process.

8. The 2017 World Anti-Doping Agency (WADA) list of banned substances does not list it. https://www.wada-ama.org/sites/default/files/resources/files/2016-09-29_-_wada_prohibited_list_2017_eng_final.pdf

9. This analysis follows the discussion in Ilundáin-Agurruza (2016, ch. 10).

10. See Lyle (2002) for a discussion of these two basic coaching styles.

11. From the Latin *ad,* "at," and *venire,* "about" in the sense of "what is to come."

12. For a comparative analysis of *mushin* and flow, see Krein and Ilundáin-Agurruza (2014). For a congruent argument for self-lessness from an enactive and situated stance, see Hutto and Ilundáin-Agurruza (2018).

13. See Ilundáin-Agurruza, Fukasawa & Takemura (2014) for parallels between pragmatism and Japanese philosophy

14. For a discussion of each of these aspects of social cognition and specific description of the experiments, see De Jaegher et al. (2010).

## REFERENCES

Abad, R. 2017. Mi currículum deportivo [My Sports CV]. http://riki-curriculum.blogspot.com/ Accessed June 18, 2017.

Ara.Cat. 2012. Emotiu record de Kilian Jornet a Stéphane Brosse: "Estaràs amb nosaltres en tots els cims." http://www.ara.cat/esports/Emotiu-record-Kilian-Jornet-Stephane-Brosse_0_723527804.html Accessed June 23, 2017.

Barzilay, Julie. Pushing the Limits: Lessons from Ultra-Endurance Athletes. http://abcnews.go.com/Health/pushing-limits-lessons-ultra-endurance-athletes/story?id=36580285 Accessed May 21, 2017

Bennett, M. and P. Hacker. 2003. *Philosophical Foundations of Neuroscience.* Malden, MA: Blackwell.

Bredo, Eric. 1994. Reconstructing Educational Psychology: Situated Cognition and Deweyian Pragmatism. *Educational Psychologist* 29(1): 23–35.

Brown, M. 2016. How Do We Keep Doping Out of Trail Running? *Outside Magazine*. https://www.outsideonline.com/2103431/how-do-we-keep-doping-out-trail-running Accessed June 30, 2017.

Butler, M. and S. Gallagher. 2018. Habits and the Diachronic Structure of the Self. In A. Altobrando, T. Niikawa and R. Stone (eds.), *The Realizations of the Self* (47–63). London: Palgrave Macmillan.

Bysted Moller, R. and V. Moller. 2015. Technology and Sport. In M. McNamee and W.J. Morgan (eds.), *Routledge Handbook of the Philosophy of Sport* (426–438). Abingdon and New York: Routledge.

Carter, Robert E. 2008. *The Japanese Arts and Self-Cultivation*. Albany: State University of New York Press.

Clarey, C.N.D. If Doping is Banned, Should Altitude Tents be Allowed for Endurance Athletes? *International Herald Tribune*. http://www.active.com/fitness/articles/if-doping-is-banned-should-altitude-tents-be-allowed-for-endurance-athletes Accessed June 24, 2017.

Cox, L. 2004. *Swimming to Antarctica: Tales of a Long Distance Swimmer*. New York: Alfred A. Knopf.

Dahl, M. 2016. The Obscure Ultra-Endurance Sport Women Are Quietly Dominating. *The Science of Us*. http://nymag.com/scienceofus/2016/09/the-obscure-endurance-sport-women-are-quietly-dominating.html Accessed October 25, 2016.

De Jaegher, H., E. Di Paolo and S. Gallagher. 2010. Can Social Interaction Constitute Social Cognition? *Trends in Cognitive Sciences* 14(10): 441–447.

Deurbrouck, J. 2012. *Anything Worth Doing: A True Story of Adventure, Friendship and Tragedy on the Last of the West's Great Rivers*. Idaho Falls, ID: Sundog Book Publishing.

Dewey. 1922. *Democracy and Education*. New York: The Macmillan Co.

Dewey. 1929. *Experience and Nature*. Chicago, IL: Open Court Pub. Co.

Dewey. 1963. *Philosophy and Civilization*. New York: Capricorn Books.

Dewey. 1980. *Art as Experience*. New York: Perigee Books.

Dewey. 1988. *Human Nature and Conduct; an Introduction to Social Psychology*. New York: Holt.

Dumons, O. 2013. Le sommet de sa vie. *Le Monde*. http://www.lemonde.fr/sport/article/2013/09/20/kilian-jornet-le-sommet-de-sa-vie_3481125_3242.html Accessed June 20, 2017.

Fodor, J. 1987. *Psychosemantics: The Problem of Meaning in the Philosophy of Mind*. Cambridge, MA: MIT Press.

Friel, J. (2003). *The Cyclist's Training Bible* (3rd ed). Boulder, CO: VeloPress.

Gallagher, S. 2009. Philosophical Antecedents to Situated Cognition. In Philip Robbins and Murat Aydede (eds.), *Cambridge Handbook of Situated Cognition* (35–50). Cambridge: Cambridge University Press.

Gallagher, S. 2013. The Socially Extended Mind. *Cognitive Systems Research* 25–26, 4–12.

Gallagher, S. 2017. *Enactivist Interventions: Rethinking the Mind*. Oxford: Oxford University Press.

Gallagher, S. and K. Miyahara. 2012. Neo-Pragmatism and Enactive Intentionality. In J. Schulkin (ed.), *Action, Perception and the Brain* (117–146). Basingstoke: Palgrave-Macmillan.
Hart, M. 2017. This Doesn't Sound Legal': Inside Nike's Oregon Project. *New York Times*. May 19. https://www.nytimes.com/2017/05/19/sports/nike-oregon-project-alberto-salazar-dathan-ritzenhein.html Accessed May 20, 2017.
Hochstetler, D. and P. Hopsicker. 2012. The Heights of Humanity: Endurance Sport and the Strenuous Mood. *Journal of the Philosophy of Sport* 39(1): 117–135.
Hochstetler, D. and P. Hopsicker. 2016. Normative Concerns for Endurance Athletes. *Journal of the Philosophy of Sport* 43(3): 335–349.
Hochstetler, D. and P. Sailors. 2015. Lead, Follow, or Get Out of the Way: A Critical Analysis of Pacing. *Journal of the Philosophy of Sport* 42(3): 349–363.
Hutto, D. 2015. Overly Enactive Imagination? Radically Re-Imagining Imagining. *The Southern Journal of Philosophy* 53: 68–89.
Hutto, D. and E. Myin 2013. *Radical Enactivism: Basic Minds without Content*. Cambridge, MA: MIT Press.
Hutto, D. and E. Myin. 2017. *Evolving Enactivism: Basic Minds Meet Content*. Cambridge, MA: MIT Press.
Hutto, D. and J. Ilundáin-Agurruza. 2018. Selfless Activity and Experience: Radicalizing Minimal Self-Awareness," with D. Hutto, Special Issue: The Relational Self—Basic Forms of Self-Awareness. *TOPOI, an International Journal of Philosophy*. https://doi.org/10.1007/s11245-018-9573-1.
Ilundáin-Agurruza, J. 2016. *Holism and the Cultivation of Excellence in Sports and Performance—Skillful Striving*. London: Routledge.
Ilundáin-Agurruza, J. 2017a. Muscular Imaginings—A Phenomenological and Enactive Model for Imagination. *Sport, Ethics and Philosophy* 11(1): 92–108.
Ilundáin-Agurruza, J. 2017b. A Different Way to Play: Holistic Sporting Experiences. In R. Scott Kretchmar (ed.), *Philosophy: Sport. Macmillan Interdisciplinary Handbooks* (319–343). Farmington Hills, MI: Macmillan.
Ilundáin-Agurruza, J., K. Fukasawa and M. Takemura. 2014. The Philosophy of Sport in Relation to Japanese Philosophy and Pragmatism. In C. Torres (ed.), *A Companion for the Philosophy of Sport* (66–82). London: Bloomsbury.
Ilundáin-Agurruza, J., K. Krein and K. Erickson. 2018. Excellence Without Mental Representation: High Performance in Risk Sports and Japanese Swordsmanshi. In M. Cappuccio (eds.), *MIT Handbook of Embodied Cognition*. Cambridge, MA: MIT Press.
Johnson, M. 2007. *The Meaning of the body: Aesthetics of Human Understanding*. Chicago, IL: University of Chicago Press.
Jornet Burgada, K. 2012. Un instante es todo lo que separa a la felicidad del dolor. *Desnivel.com*. http://desnivel.com/alpinismo/kilian-jornet-un-instante-es-lo-que-separa-la-felicidad-y-el-dolor Accessed June 24, 2017.
Krein, K. and J. Ilundáin-Agurruza, 2017. High-level Enactive and Embodied Cognition in Expert Sport Performance. *Sport, Ethics and Philosophy* 11(3): 370–384.
Krein, K. and J. Ilundáin-Agurruza. 2014. An East-West Comparative Analysis of *Mushin* and Flow. In G. Priest and D. Young (ed.), *Philosophy and the Martial Arts* (139–164). London and New York: Routledge.

Lally, R. 2013. Deweyan Pragmatism and Self-Cultivation. In R. Lally, D. Anderson and J. Kaag (eds.), *Pragmatism and the Philosophy of Sport* (175–198). London: Lexington Books.

Lally, R. 2013. Introduction. In R. Lally, D. Anderson and J. Kaag (eds.), *Pragmatism and the Philosophy of Sport* (1–16). London: Lexington Books.

Lyle, J. 2002. *Sports Coaching Concepts: A Framework for Coaches' Behaviour* (156–164). London, New York: Routledge.

MacArthur, E. 2005. *Taking on the World: A Sailor's Extraordinary Solo Race Around the Globe.* New York: McGraw-Hill.

MacIntyre, A.1984. *After Virtue: a Study in Moral Virtue.* 2nd ed. Notre Dame, IN: University of Notre Dame.

Messner, R. 2014. *My Life at the Limit.* Seattle, WA: Mountaineers Books.

McNamee, M. 2008. *Sports, Virtues and Vices: Morality Plays.* London: Routledge.

Murakami, H. 2008. *What I Talk about When I Talk About Running: A Memoir.* New York: Alfred K. Knopf.

N.A. 2014. Ricardo Abad abandona el reto de 50 'ironman' en 50 días seguidos [Ricardo Abad abandons the challenge of 50 'Ironman' in 50 days in a row] http://www.marca.com/2014/09/24/mas_deportes/deportes_aventura/1411583398.html Accessed June 23, 2017.

Ortega y Gasset, J. 2008. Hombre y Circumstancia. In *Obras Completas* (499–511), Vol. VIII. Madrid: Taurus. https://ortegaygasset.edu/publicaciones/obrascompletas/#1530530017879-386cca2e-48a6.

Piedrabuena, C. 2012a. Kilian Jornet: Soy una persona que tiene mucho miedo en la montaña y busco mucho la seguridad. [I am a person who really fears the mountain and seeks safety] *Mundo Deportivo.* http://www.mundodeportivo.com/20120529/mas-deporte/summits-of-my-life-kilian-jornet_54300860865.html Accessed June 27, 2017.

Piedrabuena, C. 2012b. Kilian Jornet: Para mí, el deporte es el medio para estar en la montaña [For me Sport is the means to be in the mountain]. *Mundo Deportivo.* http://www.mundodeportivo.com/20120509/mas-deporte/kilian-jornet-esqui-de-montana_54291356656.html Accessed June 27, 2017.

Sheets-Johnstone, M. 2009. *The Corporeal Turn: An Interdisciplinary Reader.* Exeter: Imprint Academic.

Shusterman, R. 2008. *Body Consciousness: A Philosophy of Mindfulness and Somaesthetics.* New York: Cambridge Uni. Press.

Slocum, J. 1956. *Sailing Alone Around the World.* New York: Dover Publications.

Uexküll, J.V. 2010. *A Foray into the Worlds of Animals and Humans: With A Theory of Meaning.* Minneapolis, MN: University of Minnesota Press.

Varela, F., E. Thompson and E. Rosch. 1991. *The Embodied Mind.* Cambridge, MA & London: MIT Press.

Wallace, J. 2009. *Norms and Practices.* Ithaca and London: Cornell University Press.

Yuasa, Y. 1993. *The Body, Self-Cultivation, and Ki-Energy.* Albany, NY: State University of New York Press.

*Chapter 8*

# "The Will to Believe," the Will to Win, and the Problem of Self-Transcendence

Jeffrey Fry

## INTRODUCTION

During an episode of "The Moth Radio Hour," Peter Sagal (2014), host of National Public Radio's popular "Wait Wait . . . Don't Tell Me," recounts the time that he guided blind runner William Greer during the 2013 Boston Marathon. As it happened, Greer struggled on this particular day. This was especially apparent when they reached the Newton Hills, a point about 17½ miles into the fabled 26.2-mile test of endurance. Greer was reduced to walking up Heartbreak Hill (also referred to as "Heartbreak Hell"), the most famous of the Newton Hills.[1] Nevertheless, Greer kept going. As they approached the final mile, Greer told Sagal that he believed that he would have to walk to the finish line. In response, Sagal encouraged him to run this climactic part of the race if he could. As they made a turn and headed into the last mile of the race, Greer suddenly surged ahead of Sagal. After they crossed the finish line, Sagal had to tell Greer to stop, whereupon Greer collapsed. As they wended their way from the finish line, Sagal heard a loud noise. When he turned, he saw white smoke. He then heard a second explosion. It was the Boston Marathon bombings. The blasts had occurred with the race clock showing four hours and nine minutes. Greer and Sagal had finished in about four hours and five minutes, not long before the explosions. Had they not run the last mile of the race, they might have been caught up in the bombings.

Sagal notes of Greer, "He ran that last mile. He didn't want to. But he did it."[2] Alluding to Winston Churchill's line, "If you're going through hell, keep going," Sagal says that "William Greer of Austin, Texas, blind runner, was going through hell, and he kept going."

This true story captures salient points about participation in endurance sport. Greer's running of the 2013 Boston Marathon required persistence over an extended period of time in the face of suffering. He went through hell, so to speak, and kept going. He did what at times seemed could not be done.

In keeping with this idea of strenuosity and sport, this chapter explores the relevance of the writings of American pragmatist philosopher and psychologist William James for endurance sport. Scattered throughout James' writings are references to strenuosity, both in general terms and in specific connection to sporting activities. James saw value in the strenuous life, though he believed that we habitually operate in a comfort zone below the upper reaches of our capabilities. He also explored how we tap resources that we typically hold in reserve, but which may emerge in extreme circumstances (James, 1962a). In what follows I examine not only James' writings that treat strenuosity or sporting activities directly, but also his thoughts on the will and the self, in order to shape the contours of a Jamesian-style approach to endurance sport. In the process, we may come to better understand William Greer's accomplishment in the Boston Marathon, as well as the accomplishments of other endurance athletes.

The notion of endurance sport is rich in meaning. Endurance sport has the following features. First, in order to participate in endurance sport an athlete must overcome inertia. The endurance athlete puts forth physical *effort*. This feature does not in itself distinguish endurance sport from other types of sport. Rather, what sets endurance sport apart is the extended temporal dimension typically associated with endurance sport. The endurance athlete must *sustain effort* for lengthy periods of time. A third characteristic of endurance sport sets it in yet sharper relief from other kinds of sport. This is the fact that while participating in sports such as distance running and mountain climbing, the endurance athlete must *sustain effort for long periods while enduring adversity and resistance*. The adversities include objective challenges posed by the physical environment and the athlete's physical limitations. On the experiential side, the endurance athlete must reckon with boredom, anxiety, pain and suffering, loneliness, and exhaustion. Thus, the endurance athlete must overcome various kinds of resistance.

The accomplishment of athletic goals by the endurance athlete entails a double achievement. First, the athletic accomplishes the targeted task of completing the marathon or summiting the mountain. Second, he or she explores new horizons and forges a new identity. This seemingly involves a process of self-transformation and self-transcendence.[3]

In light of the characteristic features of endurance sport, I mine James' writings for possible insights regarding the following question: How does the endurance athlete sustain effort in the face of adversity, and in the process transcend the self? I argue that James provides insights that contribute to a partial response to this question. At the same time, hesitancies, if not inconsistencies, in James' writings, create barriers to clear-cut applications of his thought to endurance sport, so that qualified assessments of his views are in order.

In part I of this chapter, I look at implications of James' (1962c) classic essay "The Will to Believe" for endurance sport. In doing so, I consider the ethical and epistemic justification of propositional beliefs and self-trust as these are implicated in endurance sport. For James, part of the pragmatic justification of belief is its efficacy in helping realize desired ends. I examine the relevance of this approach for endurance sport.

In part II, I examine the will to win, broadly conceived as the will to accomplish athletic goals in endurance sport, such as winning an endurance race, completing a marathon, or summiting a mountain. James' account of the will forms the backdrop for this discussion. Drawing on Bricklin's (1999/1999) analysis of James' account of the will,[4] I look at how James is tempted by a passive account of attention and effort, and at how this view, in turn, alters common conceptions of the endurance athlete's expression of the will to win.

In part III, I explore James' potential contributions to resolving the problem of self-transcendence as it pertains to endurance sport. How do athletes overcome fatigue and self-doubt? How do athletes break barriers, transcend seeming limitations of the self and thereby forge new athletic identities? At first blush, this possibility might seem to border on paradox. Might James have insights that help resolve the seeming paradox of the self-surpassing self?

## PART I: SPORT AND "THE WILL TO BELIEVE"

Our first consideration is the role, including the efficacy, of faith or belief in the context of endurance sport. Participation in endurance sport is an audacious enterprise.[5] Faith is involved in the initial conception of the sporting endeavor, whether it is planning an expedition to Mount Everest or contemplating running a marathon. In some cases, the initial conception and commitment involve a *leap* of faith, given the starting point and the amount of self-transformation required to accomplish the task. In coming to one's initial intention, as well as in taking intermediate steps to the goal, one engages in acts of self-displacement to a vision of a future self (or perhaps better, selves) who can accomplish the task. Between the initial conception and intention and the accomplishment of the ultimate goal lies a gap. In practice, the athlete narrows the gap through numerous incremental steps (between each of which also lies a gap). The gaps are bridged proleptically by faith. James (1962a) states that "faith is the readiness to act in a cause the prosperous issue of which is not certified to us in advance" (90). In the end, this faith will prove to be either founded or unfounded. But is it *justified*, epistemically and ethically? Further, does faith contribute to achieving the athletic goal? Finally, are the issues of justified belief and efficacious belief intertwined?

James' (1962c) classic piece "The Will to Believe" is an apology for religious faith.[6] In this work we see how James' pragmatic approach applies to the "justification *of* faith" (James, 1962c, 32; Richardson, 2007, 361).[7] In this regard, James (1962c) highlights how faith can be a necessary condition for bringing about the reality of desired states of affairs.

It is instructive to consider James' views on religious belief in light of the views of Blaise Pascal, on the one hand, and those of William Clifford, on the other. In his well-known "Wager" argument, Pascal (2002) assumes that the existence of God is intellectually undecidable. He does not attempt to prove that God exists, but rather to demonstrate that one ought to believe that God exists because it is prudent to do so. Furthermore, Pascal offers advice to the individual who is convinced by his argument, and who wants to believe, but who nevertheless does not believe that God exists. Pascal counsels that this individual should engage in religious behaviors like the devout do, and in time his or her emotional resistance may melt away and faith may flower.

William Clifford (2002) takes an opposing view. He argues that it is wrong to believe when there is insufficient evidence. To believe on grounds other than evidence contributes to one's own and others' credulity. Therefore, where the truth is intellectually undecidable, one should suspend judgment.

James (1962c) takes a middle position between the views of Pascal and of Clifford, respectively. If a proposition—such as one that stakes a religious claim—is intellectually undecidable and represents a "genuine option," then according to James one is justified in believing based on one's passional nature, that is, because one wants to believe in order to have a chance to obtain a vital good.

According to James (1962c), the genuine option has three components. First, it involves a living option. That is, both the affirmation and negation of the proposition hold some degree of credibility for the individual. Second, it is a forced option. That is, one cannot ride the fence, practically speaking. To suspend judgment is to forfeit the good in question, just as if one actively rejected the proposition in question. Third, it is a momentous option. There is a vital good at stake.

James (1962c) buttresses his argument by considering that in some cases, such as when one desires to form a relationship with another person, one may have to take a step of faith in order to create conditions that are necessary in order to fulfill the desire. In the same vein, James suggests that should ultimate reality be personal in nature, faith may be required to establish a religious relationship with that reality.

For the aspiring endurance athlete, faith is arguably also involved in the conception and launching of the effort, and in sustaining the effort required to reach both proximate and ultimate goals. Is this faith epistemically and ethically justified on James' terms? Assume that the issue of the endurance athlete's ability to achieve an athletic goal is initially intellectually undecidable. If we employ James' criteria, the question of justified belief hinges then on whether one faces a living, forced, and momentous option. First, is it a *live* option? It is always the case that one's athletic striving can be negated by injury or other limitations. But does one have some faith that the athletic goal can be realized? Second, is it a *forced* option? It is arguably so. Unless one believes—not just in a proposition, but in oneself—one will not bridge the gap between oneself and the athletic goal. Third, is the option *momentous*? To some people, participating in endurance sport holds no significance. Others, however, see it perhaps as conveying psychological and/or physical benefits and as helping maintain their identities as aspirants who thrive on the challenge of strenuous tasks.[8] In addition, the athletic goal may not be realizable at any given point in time. Rather, the timing of the pursuit of the goal may be critical. If so, this further heightens the momentousness of the option one faces.

If the criteria for a genuine option are met, as they seemingly would be in the case of some endurance athletes, then their belief in themselves would appear to be epistemically and ethically justified on James' terms. Might the legitimacy of these beliefs be further buttressed by pragmatic considerations, as James (1962c) argues is the case when considering religious belief? As previously noted, in the case of religious belief, James holds that belief in the reality of religious objects might be a necessary condition for entering into relationship with these objects, should the religious objects exist. In a similar manner, might the belief in *oneself* or *self*-trust help realize the desired athletic ends in endurance sport?

Note that in the case of the endurance athlete, the propositional belief that one can accomplish a task converges with belief in oneself.[9] Furthermore, this belief in oneself plays a dual role. First, it can serve as an indication of either one's preparedness or one's willingness to prepare for an athletic endeavor. Second, belief in oneself may be empowering, insofar as the "I can" is perhaps a necessary if not a sufficient condition of the doing. James (1962b) claims that there are cases where faith is the precondition for "subjective energy," which is the precondition for the "personal contribution," which is the precondition for the fact (97). Thus, faith lies at the foundation of establishing the fact. As James (1962b) puts it: "For again and again success depends on energy of act; energy again depends on faith that we shall not fail; and that faith in turn on the faith that we are right,—which faith thus verifies itself" (100). James' (1962b) imaginative musings on climbing in the Alps touches on the efficacy of faith during athletic endeavors.

> Suppose, for example, that I am climbing in the Alps, and have had the ill-luck to work myself into a position from which the only escape is by a terrible leap. Being without similar experience, I have no evidence of my ability to perform it successfully; but hope and confidence in myself make sure that I shall not miss my aim, and nerve my feet to execute what without those subjective emotions would perhaps have been impossible. But suppose that, on the contrary, the emotions of fear and mistrust predominate; or suppose that, having just read The Ethics of Belief, I feel it would be sinful to act upon assumption unverified by previous experience, why—then I shall hesitate so long that at last, exhausted and trembling, and launching myself in a moment of despair, I miss my foothold and roll into the abyss. In this case (it is one of an immense class) the part of wisdom is clearly to believe what one desires; for the belief is one of the indispensable preliminary conditions of the realization of its object. *There are then cases where faith creates its own verification.* (96–97)

In this example the climber takes a leap of faith, or a leap by virtue of faith.[10]

But is it necessary to justify the endurance athlete's self-trust by meeting the requirements of James' genuine option? Perhaps not. We often conduct our practical affairs in the absence of overwhelming evidence that we will succeed in our efforts. Nevertheless, James provides a response to Clifford's concerns regarding believing on insufficient evidence. This may have special relevance for the endurance athlete, given that the endurance athlete *often* commits himself or herself to achieving a goal whose attainability is uncertain. Furthermore, some justification may be appropriate given that an endurance athlete may be making a significant commitment of time and resources to the sport.

Even if we can justify the endurance athlete's belief that he or she is capable of accomplishing an athletic goal, this does not in itself justify ethically the expenditure of effort.[11] A commitment to endurance sport requires the dedication of time and resources that could be dedicated to other tasks. In addition, endurance sport can be dangerous for the participant. Given these factors, endurance sport may be viewed by some people as a selfish enterprise.[12] Endurance sport is not unique in this regard. Virtuosity in any area of performance requires sustained commitment and effort. Furthermore, many occupations have objective health hazards. The question is whether the hazards involved in endurance sport result from pursuing trivial or gratuitous endeavors, or whether they arise while engaging in worthy pursuits.[13] As James might ask, is something momentous at stake? It isn't obvious that participation in sport is, *a priori*, to be disqualified from the field of worthy endeavors. Given this, each case should be considered on an individual basis.

## PART II: THE WILL TO WIN

Even if faith in oneself is a necessary condition of success in endurance sport, it is not a sufficient condition. Other factors are involved, including physical capabilities, fortuitous sporting conditions, and general good luck. In addition, sport discourse often valorizes "the will to win." But what does it mean to *will* something?

James (1890/1950b) distinguishes between willing and wishing. Both willing and wishing involve desire. However, willing differs from wishing in that willing entails belief in the possibility of obtaining the desired end (486). James (1890/1950b) writes: "If with the desire there goes a sense that attainment is not possible, we simply *wish*; but if we believe that the end is in our power, we *will* that the desired feeling, having, or doing shall be real; and real it presently becomes, either immediately upon the willing or after certain preliminaries have been fulfilled" (486).

According to James (1890/1950b), many of our actions occur without the accompaniment of robust volition. "Ideo-motor" actions are carried out on almost automatic pilot. When motor ideas arise they are automatically accompanied by a tendency toward motor activity. If they do not meet resistance from contrary ideas, the activity will typically be carried out (522–528). James (1890/1950b) writes that "consciousness is *in its very nature impulsive*" (526). In terms of sport in general, this feature of ideas may have particular relevance in the case of those who reach high levels of expertise, or for those who, for at least brief periods, experience the condition known as "flow" (Csikszentmihalyi, 2008).[14]

Ideas have neural correlates that are central to carrying out the action. But James is perplexed about the metaphysical relationship between motor ideas and the brain. As James (1890/1950) puts it, "the mysterious tie between the thought and the motor centers" occurs "in a way which we cannot even guess at" (564).

When the individual harbors conflicting ideas the feeling of effort comes into play. Effort is a function of resistance. This conflict may be resolved by a fiat and consent. Ultimately, James holds that it is a mystery as to how this process unfolds. But James' analysis of conflicting ideas may shed light on Peter Sagal's (2014) perhaps initially perplexing claims that: (1) William Greer didn't want to run the last mile of the Boston Marathon, and (2) Greer finished the Boston Marathon because he wanted to. In some sense, both claims were likely true, insofar as he harbored conflicting ideas. This conflict was resolved in favor of running.

At the heart of James' conception of the will is the notion of attention. The exercise of the will consists of sustaining one's attention on an idea or keeping that idea in play. James (1890/1950b) writes:

> *The essential achievement of the will, in short, when it is most 'voluntary,' is to ATTEND to a difficult object and hold it fast before the mind.* The so-doing is the *fiat*; and it is a mere physiological incident that when the object is thus attended to, immediate motor consequences should ensue. (561).

As James (1890/1950b) otherwise succinctly puts it: "Effort of attention is thus the essential phenomenon of will" (562). Elsewhere James (1890/1950b) adds that it is "the strain of attention" that "is the fundamental act of will" (564). The individual who has a strong will is one who exhibits "resolute effort of attention" (James, 1890/1950b, 563–564). When the "attention is not quite complete," "express consent," "a subjective experience sui generis," may also come into play. But at this point we again enter the realm of mystery (James, 1890/1950b, 568).

What potential implications do James' thoughts on the will have for endurance sport? Endurance sport is often experienced as grueling. To the extent that this is the case, it would appear that the feeling of effort would be pervasive, notwithstanding periods of "flow," or times when second, third, or fourth wind kick in like moments of grace.[15] If we adopt James' view that was just explored, through much of the experience the challenge for the endurance athlete will be to maintain attention and to consent to motor ideas conducive to accomplishment of the task at hand. At one level then, the will to win is realized in the effort of focused attention and consent.

But can we control how much will to win we have? This brings us to the question of free will. James was ambivalent about free will. At times James struggled with the prospect of determinism.[16] Yet at other times James opted for free will on *ethical grounds* (James 1890/1950b, 573). In doing so James once again exhibited a pragmatic bent.

In the *Principles of Psychology*, James (1890/1950b) claims that the issue of free will hinges centrally on whether we can control the amount of effort or attention that we put forth. He also says that it *seems* that this condition is met. But he holds that whether or not this is *actually* the case cannot be determined by psychology (571–573).

Bricklin (2015), however, argues that there are other aspects of James' writings that bring his ambivalence about the will to the fore and complicate his desire to maintain an active center of willing and freedom of the will. Consider the following vignette from James (1890/1950b), which, as he put it, "seems to me to contain in miniature form the data for an entire psychology of volition" (525). In order to preserve the integrity of the vignette, it is necessary to quote at length.

> We know what it is to get out of bed on a freezing morning in a room without a fire, and how the very vital principle within us protests against the ordeal. Probably most persons have lain on certain mornings for an hour at a time unable to brace themselves to the resolve. We think how late we shall be, how the duties of the day will suffer; we say, "I *must* get up, this is ignominious," etc.; but still the warm couch feels too delicious, the cold outside too cruel, and the resolution faints away and postpones itself again and again just as it seemed on the verge of bursting the resistance and passing over into the decisive act. Now how do we *ever* get up under such circumstances? If I may generalize from my own experience, we more often than not get up without any struggle or decision at all. We suddenly find that we *have* got up. A fortunate lapse of consciousness occurs; we forget both the warmth and the cold; we fall into some revery connected with the day's life, in the course of which the idea flashes across us, "Hollo! I must lie here no longer"—an idea which at that lucky instant awakens no contradictory or paralyzing suggestions, and consequently produces immediately its appropriate motor effects. It was our acute consciousness of both the warmth and the cold during the period of struggle, which paralyzed our activity and kept our idea of rising in the condition of *wish* and not of *will*. The moment these inhibitory ideas ceased, the original idea exerted its effects. (James, 1890/1950b, 524–525)

Notice certain salient features of this account. First, the individual in question is caught between conflicting ideas of either staying in bed or getting out of bed. This is followed by a "lapse of consciousness." After this the idea of getting out of bed arises without contradiction. This idea "produces immediately its appropriate motor effects."

Perhaps James' account of getting out of bed on a cold morning has an apt parallel in the long-distance runner's training regimen. Getting started on a cold morning requires at least a partial resolution of conflicting ideas. At a certain point one falls into a rhythm that approximates ideo-motor action. Later, as the runner's energy wanes, the task becomes effortful in a robust sense. Contrasting ideas fill the mind. This now becomes a test of maintaining attention on the task at hand. Furthermore, for the endurance athlete, this involves the challenge of prolonging this attention over extended periods of time. As James (1962a) says regarding "human energizing": "How to keep it at an appreciable maximum? How not to let the level lapse? That is the great problem" (220).

But Jonathan Bricklin (1999/1999) offers a provocative analysis of James' "meditation" on getting out of bed on a cold morning. The analysis reveals tensions in James' thought and calls into question both the active sense of attention and free will understood in James' terms. Bricklin (1999/1999) notes James' account of thoughts without a thinker (79–80). This is James' (1890/1950a) account of consciousness bereft of an underlying thinking substance, as when James discusses the possibility that the "stream of *Sciousness* pure and simple" is "the *Thinker*" (304). On this view, thoughts arise, and thinking occurs. Furthermore, as we have seen, according to James thoughts have an automatic impulsion toward action. Given these claims, problems for free will already emerge. In addition, however, James' story of getting up in the morning involves a decision that is no decision. An idea of getting up arises after "a lapse of consciousness." The idea arises, no longer meets a resisting idea, and carries out its automatic impulsion toward action. According to Bricklin (1999/1999, 92), insofar as we restrict ourselves to introspection, "neither attention or 'express consent' to the reality of what is attended to' can be proven to be an active original force." "Direct experience" is consistent with a passive account of attention (Bricklin, 1999/1999, 92).

Bricklin (1999/1999, 86–89) holds that James' thoughts on getting out of bed anticipate the work of Benjamin Libet.[17] Libet (1999/1999) (and others) demonstrated in an experimental setting that activity (the "readiness potential" that signals the onset of an action) in the supplementary motor cortex of the brain actually precedes awareness of the intention to initiate the action by hundreds of milliseconds. Rather than initiating the action, the conscious awareness follows upon the onset of the action. Based on this discovery, Libet (1999/1999) claimed that we do not have free will, but rather an ability "to block or veto the process, so that no act occurs" (52). That is, we are not free to initiate the action, but we can stop the action from occurring. Libet (1999/1999) acknowledges that one might claim that the impulse to stop the action would itself be preceded by yet another readiness potential, which would nullify the freedom to block the action. In response, Libet suggests that the "conscious veto," as a "*control* function," "may *not* require or be the direct result of preceding unconscious processes" (53).

In *The Principles of Psychology*, James (1890/1950b) suggests that even when ideas arise impersonally, free will may consist in our ability to select from among them the ideas that we attend to. This would be, in some respects, akin to Libet's blocking of an action. However, Bricklin (1999/1999) adds a further challenge. He suggests that James' meditation on the will and other writings support a "passive model of attention" (91–93). That is, attention is just another idea that arises impersonally (91). We do not know how long the span of attention will last (90). Furthermore, Bricklin claims that James' additional consideration of consent adds nothing to attention, but rather threatens to trail off in an "infinite regress" (90).

According to Bricklin (1999/1999), insofar as James restricted himself to his claims about the limitations of psychology, and did not introduce ethical concerns, the logical conclusion of James' reflections on volition was neither freedom nor determinism, but rather indeterminism (97). As Bricklin (1999/1999) puts it: "What we believe to be acts of will are automatic reactions to stimuli of unascertainable origin" (97).

If Bricklin's account of the passive model of attention is the correct view, its implications for the conception of endurance sport are significant. Common intuitions about the will to win are overturned. The fiat is simply the resolution of conflicting ideas that takes place on impersonal terms. The notion of the endurance athlete who exhibits a will to win as an "active, original force" must be relinquished.

Bricklin poses a significant challenge to James. But there is a further complication when one attempts to propose a Jamesian framework for understanding endurance sport. This brings us to a final problem. In light of Bricklin's challenge to will as an "active, original force," can we make sense of the idea of self-transcendence in endurance sport? Furthermore, does James provide any resources for making sense of this notion? That is, given (on Bricklin's reading) James' deflationary account of will, and of thoughts without a transcendent Thinker, can we make sense of the notion of self-transcendence, and if so, how?

## PART III: THE PROBLEM OF SELF-TRANSCENDENCE

What is the problem of self-transcendence? The issue may be framed by posing another question. How, if at all, does the self succeed in surpassing itself? This postulated bootstrapping process might seem initially to be ungrounded.

To respond to this problem we must address two issues. First, we must ascertain what James means by "self." This matter is complicated or perhaps enriched by the fact that James has multiple understandings of what the self is. Second, we must then directly respond to the issue of how we propel ourselves from a present state of performance to one of improvement. How do we break through barriers in order to accomplish this? How did William Greer overcome resistance and complete the Boston Marathon?

In the *Principles of Psychology,* James (1850/1950a) identifies "the material Self," "the social Self," the spiritual Self, and "the pure Ego" (292–305). The "pure Ego" receives scant attention in James's account of the self in *The Principles of Psychology,* and as a result I will not devote further attention to it here. That leaves us with the material, social, and spiritual senses of self to consider. Of these three, the spiritual self poses particular issues.

In general terms, the notion of the self is broadly encompassing. James (1890/1950a) writes:

> *In its widest possible sense*, however, *a man's Self is the sum total of all that he* CAN *call his*, not only his body and his psychic powers, but his clothes and his house, his wife and children, his ancestors and friends, his reputation and works, his lands and horses, and yacht and bank account. All these things give him the same emotions. If they wax and prosper, he feels triumphant; If they dwindle and die away, he feels cast down,—not necessarily in the same degree for each thing, but in much the same way for all. (291–292)

The first particular notion of the self is the material self or "me." Among its constituents are my body, my clothing, my family, and my possessions (James, 1890/1950a, 291–292).

The second notion of self that James (1890/1950a) identifies is the social self. This consists of the way that others understand us. James (294) states:

> Properly speaking, a man has as many social selves as there are individuals who recognize him and carry an image of him in their mind. But as these individuals who carry the images naturally fall into classes, we may practically say that he has as many different social selves as there are distinct social groups of persons about whose opinion he cares. (James, 1890/1950a, 294)

The third notion of self is the spiritual self. It consists of dispositions and capabilities and is what we think of as the active center of the self. Again James (1890/1950a) writes:

> By the Spiritual Self, so far as it belongs to the Empirical ME, I mean a man's inner or subjective being, his psychic faculties, or dispositions, taken concretely.... These psychic dispositions are the most enduring and intimate part of the self, that which we most verily seem to be. We take a purer self-satisfaction when we think of our ability to argue and discriminate, of our moral sensibility and conscience, of our indomitable will, than when we survey any of our other possessions. (296)

Again, finally:

> Now, *what is the self of all other selves?*

> Probably all men would describe it in much the same way up to a certain point. They would call it the *active* element in all consciousness; saying that whatever qualities a man's feelings may possess, or whatever content his thoughts may include, there is a spiritual something in him which seems to *go out* to meet these qualities, whilst they seem to *come in* to be received by it. It is that which

welcomes or rejects. It presides over the perception of sensations, and by giving or withholding its assent it influences the movements they tend to arouse. It is the home of interest,—not the pleasant or painful, not even pleasure or pain, but that within us to which pleasure or pain, the pleasant and the painful, speak. It is the source of effort and attention, and the place from which emanate fiats of the will. (James, 1890/1950a, 297–298)

Insofar as our bodies are transformed and our physical capabilities are thereby enhanced, or insofar as we acquire possessions, our material selves are transcended. There is perhaps no inherent paradox here. Furthermore, insofar as others' opinions of us change, including those regarding our athletic prowess, no formidable obstacle exists to transformations of the social self. But how does our spiritual self—the self that James says is connected to our "indomitable will"—surpass itself, particularly given the passive model of attention? How does one break through barriers during times of fatigue and self-doubt?

A key to resolving the apparent paradox of the self-surpassing self may lie in James' (1962a) "The Energies of Men." If we take seriously the passive account of attention and the challenge that it presents to free will, then perhaps it is other aspects of the self than the spiritual self that are the "dynamogenic agents" or "stimuli for unlocking what would otherwise be unused reservoirs of individual power" (James, 1962a, 231). In "The Energies of Men," James (1962a) asks, "in the fluctuations of which all men feel in their own degree of energizing, to what are the improvements due, when they occur" (222). James (1962a) responds: "Either some unusual stimulus fills them with emotional excitement, or some unusual idea of necessity induces them to make an extra effort of will. *Excitements, ideas, and efforts*, in a word, are what carry us over the dam" (222). While James (1962a) writes that "ascetic discipline" (229) plays an empowering role, the extent to which other factors are key is striking. These include "duty, the example of others, and crowd pressure and contagion" (James, 1962a, 223). These are factors outside the confines of the spiritual self. To some extent they implicate the social self. But this means that the self is not an isolated self.

What was the dynamogenic impetus that helped William Greer draw on reserves that enabled him to complete the Boston Marathon? It was, at least in part, the crowds who lined the miles of streets and applied their "bullying" encouragement.[18] It was the women of Wellesley College who raised a chorus of support. It was the people who cheered him on to the finish line as Greer turned into the last mile of the Boston Marathon. And it was Peter Sagal. They were all both aspects of Greer's social self and agents of grace.

The transformative power of social grace is found elsewhere in sport. Indeed, it is nearly ubiquitous. As I have recounted elsewhere (Fry, 2011), mountain climber Beck Weathers (2001) experienced his own moments of grace that saved his life on Mt. Everest during the deadly climbing season of 1996. After being left for dead during a blizzard on the South Col of Everest, he recovered consciousness and had a vision of his family. In those moments he realized that he would either get up or die. He stood up and walked to high camp. Others helped him off the mountain. Though much more dramatic, Weathers' experience is reminiscent in some ways of James' meditation on getting up out of bed on a cold morning. In Weathers' case, his internalized social self tapped a reservoir of energy, and his spiritual self, that seeming center of attention that receives and goes out into the world, found that he got up.

## CONCLUSION

James account of the will is complex and multi-faceted. Thus, its relevance for endurance sport is also multi-layered. In part I of this chapter, I showed that for James, the will to believe enters into the epistemic and ethical justification of belief. In part this is due to the efficacy of belief. I suggested that James' "justification of belief" might have applications to endurance sport. Indeed, belief may be a precondition of accomplishing the endurance athlete's goals.

In part II, I showed that for James, willing is related especially to sustaining attention. Effort is involved insofar as ideas are met with resistant, contrary ideas. This too has applications to the endurance athlete insofar as he or she entertains conflicting ideas about participation. Drawing on Bricklin, we saw a tension in James between active and passive accounts of attention and waffling about free will. The surprising implications of James' deflationary account of the will were that the endurance athlete does not exert will to win as an active force.

In part III, I analyzed the problem of self-transcendence and the endurance athlete. The initial paradox of the self-surpassing self of the endurance athlete was resolved by drawing on James' multiple senses of self. In particular, I suggested that the social self comes to the aid of the spiritual self to resolve the paradox.

This account of James and the will is in one sense deflationary, insofar as it uncovers and underlines a passive account of the will. However, in another sense it is expansive, in that it highlights the endurance athlete's indebtedness to the social self and to grace. In the final analysis, at least on this interpretation of aspects of James' thought, the will to win is distributed, and so is our freedom.

Finally, we return to William Greer. How did he keep going? The mystery has a partial resolution. On this reading of James' account of the will and the self, belief and energy ignited by his social self, help explain how William

Greer, who both did and didn't want to run the Boston Marathon, went through hell and kept going.

## ACKNOWLEDGMENTS

I would like to thank Elizabeth N. Agnew and the editor Doug Hochstetler for their comments on this chapter. I am grateful for the opportunity that I had to present a version of this chapter at the joint Conference of the British Philosophy of Sport Association and European Association for the Philosophy of Sport, April 2017.

## NOTES

1. For this information about the Boston Marathon course (including a reference to "heartbreak hell"), see "2006 Boston Marathon; The Course"; "The course: Fun, then sweat, then heartbreak hell," boston.com Sports
http://archive.boston.com/marathon/course/stage3.htm, retrieved January 30, 2017.

2. Earlier Sagal (2014) said that Greer had completed the Boston Marathon "because he wanted to do it." The seeming conflict between saying Greer did and didn't want to do it is perhaps addressed by James' notion of conflicting ideas within the individual.

3. Anderson and Lally (2004, 21) refer to "self-revision." Of course, failure to achieve an athletic goal may also lead to self-transformation, and not necessarily in a negative way. For example, an athlete may learn humility. For an example of this, see the moving portrayal of the fall and redemption of former National Football League quarterback Ryan Leaf in the ESPN E:60 documentary on Leaf's football career and subsequent life, which included time in prison. I am indebted to Doug Hochstetler for encouraging me to think about what happens to identity and self-transformation when one fails to meet one's goals.

4. See also Bricklin (2015).

5. I wish to acknowledge inspiration here from former U.S. President Barack Obama's book title, *The Audacity of Hope: Thoughts on Reclaiming the American Dream* (2006).

6. For a critical analysis of James' approach to justification of belief, see Blackburn (2005).

7. James (1907/1955) writes that the "pragmatic method" involves an "*attitude of looking away from first things, principles, 'categories,' supposed necessities; and of looking towards last things, fruits, consequences, facts*" (47).

8. For an apology for endurance sport, see Anderson and Lally (2004).

9. Note that this account does not presuppose any particular explanation of how beliefs are instantiated. This account is consistent with both reductionistic and nonreductionistic accounts of the mind.

10. Of course it is possible that faith is a mere epiphenomenal correlate of the leap. If so, any efficacy attributed to faith would be an unfounded postulate of folk psychology.

11. For an enlightening approach to meeting ethical requirements while participating in endurance sport, see Hochstetler and Hopsicker (2016). Fry (2004) offers caveats regarding investing too much of our lives in sport.

12. On some of the sacrifices associated with mountain climbing, see Coffey (2003).

13. Again, for a defense of the value of endurance sport, see Anderson and Lally (2004).

14. See Csikszentmihaly (2008, 96–100). See also Anderson and Lally (2004) on Csikszentmihalyi, flow, and sport.

15. On the experience of these further iterations of the phenomenon of "second wind," see (James, 1962a, 216–217).

16. On James' wrestling with free will and determinism, see Richardson (2007).

17. See, e.g., Libet (1999/1999).

18. On the notion of "bullying-treatment," see James (1962a, 222).

## REFERENCES

Anderson, D.R. and R. Lally. (2004). Endurance sport. *Streams of William James*, 6(2), 17–21.

Blackburn, S. (2005). *Truth: A guide*. Oxford, UK: Oxford University Press.

Bricklin, J. (1999/1999). A variety of religious experience: William James and the non-reality of free will. In B. Libet, A. Freeman, & K. Sutherland (Eds.), *The volitional brain: Towards a neuroscience of free will* (77–98). Thorverton, UK: Imprint, Academic. Reprint from *Journal of Consciousness Studies*, 6(8–9), 1999, 77–98.

Bricklin, J. (2015). *The illusion of will, self, and time: William James's reluctant guide to enlightenment*. Albany, NY: State University of New York Press.

Clifford, W.K. (2002). The ethics of belief. In David Shatz (Ed.), *Philosophy and faith: A philosophy of religion reader* (429–433). Boston, MA: McGraw-Hill.

Coffey, Maria. (2003). *Where the mountain casts its shadow: The dark side of extreme adventure*. New York, NY: St. Martin's Press.

Csikszentmihalyi, M. (2008). *Flow: The psychology of optimal experience*. New York, NY: Harper Perennial Modern Classics.

Fry, J.P. (2004). Sports and "the fragility of goodness." *Journal of the Philosophy of Sport*, 31, 34–46.

Fry, J.P. (2011). Making a comeback. *Sport, Ethics and Philosophy*, 5(1), 4–20.

Hochstetler, D. and Hopsicker, P.M. (2016). Normative concerns for endurance athletes. *Journal of the Philosophy of Sport*, 43(3), 335–349.

James, W. (1890/1950a). *The principles of psychology*, vol. 1. New York, NY: Dover Publications, Inc.

James, W. (1890/1950b). *The principles of psychology*, vol. 2. New York, NY: Dover Publications, Inc.

James, W. (1907/1955). Pragmatism. In R.B. Perry (Ed.), *Pragmatism and four essays from the meaning of truth* (17–153). Cleveland, OH: Meridian Books/The World Publishing Company.
James, W. (1962a). The energies of men. In R.B. Perry (Ed.), *Essays on faith and morals* (216–237). New York, NY: The New American Library, Inc.
James, W. (1962b). The sentiment of rationality. In R.B. Perry (Ed.), *Essays on faith and morals* (62–110). New York, NY: The New American Library, Inc.
James, W. (1962c). The will to believe. In R.B. Perry (Ed.), *Essays on faith and morals* (32–62). New York, NY: The New American Library, Inc.
Libet, B. (1999/1999). Do we have free will. In B. Libet, A. Freeman, & K. Sutherland (Eds.), *The volitional brain: Towards a neuroscience of free will* (47–57). Thorverton, UK: Imprint, Academic. Reprint from *Journal of Consciousness Studies*, 6(8–9), 1999, 47–57.
Obama, B. (2006). *The audacity of hope: Thoughts on reclaiming the American dream*. New York, NY: Crown Publishers.
Pascal, B. (2002). The wager. In David Shatz (Ed.), *Philosophy and faith: A philosophy of religion reader* (474–476). Boston, MA: McGraw-Hill.
Richardson, R.D. (2007). *William James in the maelstrom of American modernism*. Boston, MA: Mariner Books/Houghton Mifflin Company.
Sagal, P. (recorded February 10, 2014). Keep going; The moth: True stories told live. http://player.themoth.org/#/?actionType=ADD_AND_PLAY&storyId=298, retrieved January 30, 2017.
Weathers, B. (2001). *Left for dead: My journey home from Everest*. New York, NY: Dell Publishing.

*Chapter 9*

# On Meaning and Motive in Endurance Sport

## *An Experiential Romp through the Grand Whys*

Scott Tinley

"Everybody wants to be an endurance athlete," I imagine a conversation between myself and other colleagues; some of us having more or less experience as endurance athletes and/or researchers of the topic. "That's what matters in the current world of physical culture. What gives you cred on the cocktail party circuit are the numbers on your bumper stickers. People let you merge into their lane if they see *26.2*, more so than *13.1*."

What does my colleague know, I wonder? She has only completed six marathons and one half Ironman-distance triathlon. "My good woman," I reply in jest, "has your ideological approach to endurance sports been reduced to fractions of a shifting whole? What happens when some new kind of summation takes hold and the numbers on the back of your vehicle reflect something all-together different? Can you pull them off the chrome as fast as you can shift your training program and philosophical positions?"

She asks if I can offer a more cogent philosophical argument explaining the postmodern popularity of endurance sports. "What is the basis," she parried, "to why people pay for pain, and then brag about it? Why did *you* purposely embrace all that discomfort for so many years?"

I had no sustainable argument then.

Now, some years later, my intellectual travels and travails reconstituted in synch with my memories of fifteen years as a professional triathlete, I am only slightly closer to being able to explain the popularity of endurance sports. Just when I think I have the answer something changes—a new champion, new technology, new media platforms, new sponsors; the world of endurance sports appears directly linked to the shifting sands of popular thought, culture, science, and economy. Yet American minds have circuitously been informing some explanation for well over a century. William James (1962) discussed the notion of "leveling" in his essay, *What Makes a Life Significant*. Aren't endurance athletes constantly being *leveled* by the elements, their bodies, and the competition . . . the necessary and ubiquitous details of living? Emerson (1981) suggests in his essay, *Circles*, "the key to every man is his thought" (230). What endurance athlete has not returned from a long run or ride feeling fuller and closer to his existentiality, the benefit of time to think? In addition, there is Thoreau's (2012) *deliberateness*. There is Sheehan's (1978) rift on *playfulness*. There is Murakami's (2008) effort to connect his complicated *physicality/creativity connection* within the simple act of running.

I want to know why all the modern fuss over endurance sport. However, not at the risk of losing its wonderment-hold on me as I enter my fiftieth year running, and swimming, and riding my bike around the block. Dewey (in Williams, 1951) suggests, "The local is the only universal upon all that art builds" (330). My motive was clear enough to lace up a pair of running shoes in the rain today, to enjoin that puddle-wonderful world. My training partner rolled over and went back to sleep. We are both local but could not find our universal motive today. Perhaps tomorrow.

This chapter is an effort to take but a sampling of American philosophy and seek what universal might exist in explaining the growing popularity of endurance sports in the new millennium.

## THE QUEST THEORY OR ENDURANCE SPORTS AS HERO MAKER

The frontiers have been discovered, the Wild West tamed, the deep seas explored, and at least one of the planets in our solar system slated for soil sampling before the first stucco-sided cul-de-sac is built in a faux-colonial architectural motif. These are difficult times for mountain men and hunter-gatherers; the jobs are scarce, the rivers choked. Colonial battles have lost their luster. So we turn to endurance sports to fulfill our behavioral drive to explore and discover; to test and conquer and confront our existential intent. To feel heroic. My colleague's queries, if not her challenge, suggest that the reasons and motivations for running three or thirty-three miles have much more depth than we have been able to substantiate in dialogue or data. James (1962) tells us that a life lived in service of ideals can be significant particularly when rife with "dogged endurance and insensibility to danger" (295). However, what ancient folkloric-heroic values are to be seen in the athlete who goes off in search of dragons or great mountains simply because they are there? The fruits of their ventures may not be as obvious as running into a burning building to save a puppy but they can and do inspire us with their operationalized idealism.

The Grand Why of modern endurance athlete's motive reflects a human species that, at face value, appears to have pushed back against the mid-twentieth-century popular restraint. *Less-is-more*, our parents were schooled, *you only have a fixed number of heart beats*, old school rhetoric argued, and *running was for cavemen*. Lest we forget, bradycardia (slow resting pulse) as a result of either genetics or endurance sport training, was treated with amphetamine prescriptions until the late 1950s. So, to witness a refusal of that underdeveloped science, a challenge to the rhetoric that may have temporally limited our ability to connect with our somatic selves, is to celebrate what? Sports and resistance? Sport and exploration? Frank Shorter's marathon win at the 1972 Munich Olympic Games? Julie Moss crawling to second place at the 1982 Ironman Triathlon? On the other hand, would it suggest that from a physical standpoint, life for many had become too easy, too predictable . . . what might be called the *banality of somatics*.[1]

If America has but one archetypal myth, it is that of the renegade, the explorer, the man and woman willing to risk their current place in life to find that which fulfills the dream, the quest. It does not begin or end with a worldly feat of endurance for as James (1962) reminds us, "not a victory is gained . . . except upon a maybe" (369). To have the ideal, a *maybe I can do that*, is the beginning of heroism and a life worth being lived.

Start with the recent past. Many souls have been sliced open, emotional blood spilt on that island of endurance sport in search of personal *heroism*. But if some concept of hero status, quasi as it might be and attained through participation in endurance sports stands as evidence for its mass popularity, we might return to Emerson, Campbell, and Carlyle.[2] How transferable are their notions of the hero quest to our current popular application of celebrities, entertainers, event makers, and professional athletes? Emerson (1981) suggests that all mythology opens with demigods. But his *Representative Men* (Plato, Swendenborg, Montaigne, Shakespeare, Napoleon, and Goethe) were nearly to a man, intensely physical humans. "Every true man," Emerson suggests in *Self-Reliance*,[3] "is a cause, a country, and an age . . . posterity seems to follow his steps as a train of clients" (148). Still, failing modern empirical data that supports the connection of endurance sports' popularity with some notion of a need to struggle, to follow one's ideal, to use that warrior's heart where the athlete feels the need to be needed, all we have is anecdote—the local's tale as universal.

On the other hand, failing to respect if not understand the collective effort of millions of runners, swimmers, cyclists, paddlers, hikers, climbers, etc. is a failure to realize the collaborative suffrage born of personal quests reared in the unexplained sharing of that pain. Our struggle is made, motivated, and celebrated *ensemble* as one might a poem or a song, or the development of a country; each coming to it on their own but walking away in the afterglow of some unspoken aesthetic collective.[4]

I started distance running in junior high school. I was thirteen years old in 1970 and my coach was a counter-culturalist who advocated running in suede Indian moccasins rather than leather spikes. In 1970 there were no specific shoes designed to run on "the roads" which meant anything other than a designated dirt track or trail; we ran around the parks and pathways in our leather and suede footwear and heavy cotton shorts. Two miles was a distance workout. We talked about connecting to nature through the art of running if for no other reason than it seemed a different approach to the concept of physical fitness. Alternatively, perhaps those drawn to the individual sports simply lacked the eye–hand coordination standards needed to play varsity team sports. We were not channeling Thoreau specifically but our small band of runners marched quite opposite athletes drummed-up as footballers and hoopsters.

The term "jogging" had not yet entered the modern lexicon. Sometime that summer I went on vacation with my family and ended up running on the side of the road somewhere in rural New Mexico. It felt good if not right but I could never explain why at the time. Every other car stopped to ask if I was in trouble—did I need a ride? Had there been an accident? Had I committed a crime? In Gumpian fashion, I just felt like running.

The late 1960s had been a tumultuous time to go through puberty. As I understand now, my quest through the act of running was not about finding a cure for cancer, saving the whales, or stopping the war in Vietnam. I had no heroic aspirations and only wanted girls to like the skinny, pimply, pass-dropping, free throw-missing pubescent that I was.

Undeniably, there are still many of us who feel the need to submit to that call toward the physical edge—that entrancing whistle from the unknown. But why? For what are we searching or running? Moreover, how do we find it or lose it? Fiction writer, Alan Sillitoe (1959) suggested our answers to the individual and collective call have something to do with identity searches sought within societies' rents and seams. Deviant behavior, legal or not, can take us to (in)hospitable zones where the risk is not always equal to the reward. Nevertheless, we go for what might be found. Sillitoe's protagonist, Smith offers:

> I knew what the loneliness of the long distance runner running across country felt like, realizing that as far as I was concerned this feeling was the only honesty and realness there was in the world and knowing it would be no different ever, no matter what I felt at odd times, and no matter what anybody else tried to tell me. (Sillitoe, 37)

So we go to the edges of our athletic forest, unable to deny the lure, glad that there is still an opportunity to go out beyond the last houses, beyond our comfort zone to that place inside our minds and our bodies that will appear dangerous, even deadly. Or, as Thoreau (2012) suggests in his Walden chapter, Higher Laws, "I love the wild not less than the good" (369).[5]

## AESTHETIC FASHION-EMULATION THEORY

Endurance sport pundits who argue that the sporting masses simply tired of stick and ball sports might also consider another cultural turn of the sneaker sect. Late twentieth century's popularity of endurance sport, it might be argued, began with Frank Shorter's gold medal in the 1972 Munich Olympic Marathon. No American had won Modern Olympic gold in the marathon. Suddenly the wire thin, twenty-five-year-old Yale graduate was hip. Consumers wanted to have what Shorter had. If it could not be his athletic endurance, then at least it could be his athletic clothing and his choice of physical activity. Desire was fulfilled from the production side and endurance sport-as-fashion was born. Explained in later works by Jameson (1998) and Giddens (1991), the notion of identity through consumption as applied to some aspect of the rise in endurance sports' popularity is perhaps better validated simply by observing the rise in endurance sports-related companies. Phil Knight and Bill Bowerman's Blue Ribbon Sports (Nike), German-based, Dassler brothers' Puma and Adidas, and then the organic Bill Rogers and Frank Shorter endurance running brands catalyzed the idea that function could be fashionable, that running in circles was not a penance but a gift. By the mid-1970s, you could stop by the market after a run or ride[6] or a swim still wearing nylon tricot shorts or spandex and a water-resistant, breathable jacket and actually look if not feel comfortable in the badge of fitness that was your workout attire. Patterns, colors, cuts, and fabrication of running clothes bled into discussions of training regimes. A prime motive to participate in endurance sports in the 1970s and early 1980s was simply that it was a cool thing to do. Fitness and health benefits were often seen as an afterthought. There was also an attached aesthetic created and celebrated in words.

Writers such as Sheehan (1978), Murakami (2008), Bugbee (1958),[7] and John L. Parker (1978)[8] exposed a deeply existential basis that many had felt but few could explain. The popular narratives, both real and imagined, spoke of long steady athletic feats facilitating long and steady but telling pain, moments ticked off in a variable period reference, some moving so agonizingly slow that leg cramps could seem like childbirth contractions—rhythmic, ceaseless but laden with a purpose. Or perhaps the narratives of pain—reframed as thoughtful if not justifiable—were must-know topics within emerging sports culture.

Parker's (1990) protagonist in *Once a Runner*, the former collegiate miler, Quenton Cassidy, muses on which of the four laps to the mile is most difficult:

> The third lap was a microcosm, not of life, but of the Bad Times, the times to be gotten through, the no-toys-at-Christmas, sittin'-at-the-bus-station-at-midnight blues times to look back on and try to laugh about or just forget. The third lap was to be endured and endured and endured. (246–247)

Dr. George Sheehan's 1978 New York Times bestseller, *Running and Being: The Total Experience* introduced millions of runners to the notion that sport, and endurance running in particular, could be a cerebral experience. Perhaps even spiritual. "The best most of us can do," he offers, "is to be poet an hour a day" (110). Sheehan's material penned for various popular texts, failed as rigorous philosophy. But in many ways his carefully calculated and analogue texts are distinctly American in their organic relevance to what endurance athletes were doing and thinking about during the mid to late 1970s. Long run conversations inevitably fell to the oft-asked question: What would Sheehan say about *that*?

Our overarching achievements in endurance sport now appear to be contextually bound by how we perceive their material if not existential value. One person's M-dot tattoo (signifying an Ironman Triathlon finisher)[9] is another's skin cancer. For many, endurance sports bring with them their own kind of bearing, their own signature and stamp on our lives. We will not really know what that will be until we try; until you find a kind of Jamesian victory in the simple, "well, maybe I can go the distance." You might feel younger for the effort or you might finally realize that rust never sleeps and that you were caught red-handed with desires exceeding assets.

Either way, you may have a significant-life moment. Either way, the burden and blessing of success-by-excess, even if motivated by shallow, external reasons, facilitates a way of being in the physical and popular world. This may be why, as Suits (1978) asks, we submit ourselves to the *purposeful attempt to overcome unnecessary obstacles*. Why suffer through a one-hundred-mile bike ride when riding ten or fifteen or even twenty-five would be a healthier choice? Perhaps lucky are the ones who find transcendence in a 5k walk, who can access the artfulness of endurance sport by swimming five hundred yards, not five hundred days in a row. But who can say? Thoreau argues for sauntering while James suggests the occasional strenuous mood. Both are acceptable within the context of time, definition, and end result. For those who have logged decades of participation in search of something beautiful in the world of endurance sports and ended up with good ideas and great memories but health issues ranging from soft tissue loss to cardiac events, only they can tell if it was worth it. "Training for and competing in endurance sport can be threatening to human affiliation," Hochstetler and Hopsicker (2016) suggest, "when the overall sport ethos is corrupt" (341). The "corruption" they speak of extends into misguided or mistaken information in such imperatives as the risk/reward ratio inherent to endurance training and competition. Still, even the well-coached and astute athlete can be blinded by the power of immortality narratives.

## FOUNTAIN OF YOUTH THEORY

Disparity in purpose is often seen in the way adults come to play childhood games. Some of us show up to the weekend tracks and pools and parking lots loaded for bear, the drippings of week-long, corporate, cut-throat tailings on our purposeful steps. Others are happy for a few kindred minutes of coffee-conversation and a chance to wax poetic of days before gravity pulled down our waistline dreams. In between are a gazillion other twenty-one-and-older types who look to post-baccalaureate endurance sports participation for myriad reasons that are reasonably muddled. There is an attraction to return to endurance sports after college and career and kids and a mortgage. But we do not always know *where* or *how* to place our age-encumbered bodies in that early midlife term. So, the *why* is left to rise to the surface on its own, and when it does, we might not recognize it.

At twenty-five, you are still slim, fit, and competitive. At thirty-five, you are fit and competitive. At forty-five, you tell yourself that you are still competitive. But you are not sure at what. Or why. That is when your world of endurance sports gets more curious. It is hard to admit, let alone clarify, your reasons for returning to sport. We seek ways to prove our own adult involvement in physical games normally reserved for youth. We thirst for any kind of explaining pugmark of success—a finisher's T-shirt, a plastic medal, a recycled bowling trophy—just something tangible to hold and feel and place in plain view. Then we are reminded that the most popular sports-related injury each of the last ten years is from sliding into base during a softball game.

The rational mind tells us that we will not run as fast as we did in high school or swim as fluid as we did in college. But if we learned anything in those four (or six) years, it's that the effects of time only appear to be linear. The body willing, you can still bend time like you bent weekend parties into entire semesters. You are in control, you remind yourself. You are not dead.

So, you don't outwardly question this desire to be young again for the second time, to play, to compete, to win at something, if only some beer-bet with yourself to lose five pounds by the first of next month. A sport is the answer; you tell yourself without even knowing what the question was. *Yes, something athletic that makes me sweat and look good in spandex and that exorcises the office demons before I get home. I'll figure out the rest as I go. But I don't want to get hurt, sit on the bench, or otherwise try to look like I'm trying too hard.*

But somehow we are still afraid of returning as a soft child stuck in an adult's hardening body. *Act your age*, we tell ourselves, although we are not sure on what scale it is to be accounted. What is lost in translation are the meanings that sport used to give us as a kid. Is *Adult Endurance Sports* an oxymoron? A new language? A way to burn off the vicissitudes of corporate culture? Or is it a way to stop the clock for a weekend or a decade and reframe what a physical life can do for us? The answer may lie in that netherworld where sports and a style of living overlap.

Endurance sports do not happen in different dimensions from our daily lives; there is no schizophrenia, no fifty-yard split of ethos and ethic. We do not go to the crossroads to deal for our fitness and health. For many of us, it just seems natural, this physical life. Returning to sport as an adult does not mean compromising on all that is huge, permanent, and fixed. It is not an early, middle, or late-life crisis. It is just another way of living. Endurance sport is a kind of life that people choose, and life is a kind of game that people play—a Venn diagram that deserves some fun in the gray areas.

As endurance athletes, we develop these skills, these tendencies to pull down psychological barriers that rise up again in the biological. Age is a state of mind, we tell ourselves, in drowning the noise of a screaming tendon. As we ignore these smoke signals harboring things to come, we go around the track one more time, harder now because the guru-jock-of-the-month says in his or her new book that fitness is greater than health, and if we must have an addiction, then what better habit to be enslaved to? This sporting life, we are convinced, is the only life. For many of us, we could willingly allow self-deception. The only thing wrong is too much of a right thing, we tell ourselves, and had only Icarus reduced his altitude earlier.

The action-hero philosophers will tell us that life is about experiences, feelings, successes, and failures. It is the sum of smoke and deception, purpose and direction, love and hate, yingiditty-yang and you fill in the gaps. Sport is at once phenomenological and self-reflexive. It is fun to live on the edge so long as we do not go over. Why slide into base when we can keep running around them?

## SOCIALIZATION THEORY

In our naïveté of youth, our halcyon days before the weight of age tugs at our dreams and our belts, we circle the track and feel the soft rubber under our feet and smell the fresh cut grass as we temporarily enslave ourselves to the stopwatch. Each lap has meaning, we tell ourselves, each lap is quicker, deeper into our goal. But what do we really know at fourteen or eighteen or twenty-two years old? Too often our goals are more general-directing than specific-in-plan. Many of us have come to equate success with material gain, something tangible with a leather interior and a GPS to show us the way. But we also find great joy in the realization that we are learning along the way.

In our own freshman fame, in those times when we wanted things we would never get and got things that we never wanted, we just might've known that we were both passenger and pilot. While we were building a body, we were building a social life. But at seventeen or twenty-one, those things were only barely within our control—our lives flying IFR (instrument flying rules). Perhaps endurance sports helped us to figure it all out as we landed on planet adulthood. Atkinson (2008), writing of triathletes, notes that "within a mutually identified community of athletes, the ability to withstand and relish in athletic suffering is embraced as a form of group distinction" (165–166), and as Hochstetler and Hopsicker (2016) suggest, "the triathletes' desire for self-imposed pain in the leisure area binds them together as a unique social group; what we might call a unique 'pain community'" (338). But as the birthdays came closer and quicker we pined for that something still fresh and unnamable, something closer to spiritual than cellular. It was earned, we felt, through blood, sweat, years, and many more miles. But it sure would help with motivation if all my friends were doing it.

The burgeoning endurance sport of triathlon gained traction within the gluttonous mid 1980s when the economy boomed in synch with cultural narcissism (Lasch, 1979). Triathletes shoe-horned cut and trimmed figures into neon spandex and the very *idea* of endurance sports was shape-shifted from mangy-bearded, Thoreau-quoting runners and elitist, private-schooled, Euro-wannabee cyclists to something very hip and distinctly American. Born on the boggy shores of San Diego, the triple sport was originally and instinctually linked to sun, surf, and sexuality. Fittingly, one of the first time the term "triathlon" graced popular culture was in Wolfe's 1987 *Bonfire of the Vanities*, a depicture of mid-1980s New York City debauchery. This new endurance sport socialized us then and now. It felt good to find an ideology of excess that fit our lifestyle choices, but also taught us something, even if it was hard-earned humility when our bodies failed to keep up with our egos.

I remember the exact moment when I crossed the line between training for performance sake and training for training's sake, when sport had become my life but also a kind of slow dance with hubris. Oh, there had been occasional balance, but it came as two junkyard dogs circling each other. It was during the birth of our first child, my wife in the jaws of a protracted but not entirely uncomfortable labor. I pulled the doctor aside and asked him if I had time to sneak outside for a quick five-miler. I would stay on the hospital grounds. I promised. That memory haunts me still, how I had folded myself tightly into sport and that part of me was so far away from the essential cycle of life itself that the only satisfaction was an audience of one and the cackling laughter I would hear in the background could only be the devil's.

No athlete can hide forever behind the thinly veiled excuse of ignorance. At least we should know when too much might be too much. Still, if we see sport and life as one, it is a great task to distinguish the map from the territory, to differentiate a training program from a training lifestyle. Equal parts passion and pragmatism.

You see, endurance sport at any age can act as a drug. The needle slips in when you slip out of your mother's womb. There is a terrifying excitement where part of you wants to go back into the shade and the other wants to jump into the light. You tell yourself that you just do not know. How could you? Therefore, you follow your instincts to move because somehow it is born with you, the knowledge that something possessed never has the same value or pull as it does in pursuit. You might be chasing your tail but at least you are not lying in the corner.

Many of us are hooked to some degree. It is certainly not hard to extol the virtue in endurance sport. Simple, really. Bang away at the keys, chat up a stranger on a plane, or convince a relative over for Christmas dinner that endurance sport is good, that it is different; it allows us a chance to stand out. *From where*, they ask. *From here, silly. Anywhere but right here, doing nothing.* With your sport, you tell them, you can glow in the dark. And you would be right. That is the bad part of the drug—it can bend a reality on its own accord, squiggly lines on a desert horizon. Mirage goes from noun to verb. You glow when you are supposed to fade.

George Sheehan (1978), physician, writer, and 1970s running guru, gave us permission to find our metaphysical selves outside the traditional lines with suggestions such as "there (are) two types of successful fitness programs. One is rational, practical, physiological; the other nonrational, mystical, and psychological" (51). For those concerned with physiological results steeped in practical rationality, the benefits of endurance sport become measurable, obvious, and concise. But Sheehan, a master of manipulating (sometimes oblique) citations to fit his narratives, suggests a disparate contrary: "The other program is for unhappy people who find that it is life that is mindless, inconvenient, and boring" (52). Likely, many endurance athletes draw from wells born of both conscientious thought and creativity; from careful preparation and impulsive abandonment.

When we consider our Great Whys in endurance sports, statistics are our ammo and the media is our ally. Numbers never lie, we are led to believe, and neither do heroes. It is all so true because we want to believe it. Sportsmanship, camaraderie, physical health, goal attainment, self-knowledge—they are all there inside of endurance sport, neatly packaged sometimes, raw and unwieldy at others. Sport provides a constellation of possibilities, and we could be a star in our own galaxy. Oh God, it is so easy—twinkle, twinkle, and I am dating someone younger and thinner than me, another twinkle and I have a tan in December, I won my age group and another twinkle. If only I did not have this job I could've made The Show, could have stepped right into that aristocracy of fame: a fat house, a skinny spouse, the UPS driver calling me by my first name.

Go for it, endurance sport says, grab the brass ring and find yourself separated from a normal life and do not worry about separating from your old Self. A better one awaits. If you return, you are just a posttraumatic game show away from the regularity of a remote control and sixer of plain wrap generic beer. Perhaps it is not that easy to find meaning in sports if we are too busy looking extra hard—if we equate positive meaning with positive competitive results. Athletes and endurance athletics have become a fixture in our culture, socializing our youth, teaching them valuable lessons not so easily taught at home or in the classroom. It means a lot to endure physical challenges.

Still, sport thrills us like few institutions can, often overshadowing theater, the arts, music, and war as the chosen form of entertainment. Not since the Roman Empire has sport played such a role in how we live our aging lives. Is it because commercial sport remains the last form of popular culture in which the ending is still a mystery? Or is it that we lust for something memorable?

## THE MEMORY THEORY OR RITUAL, RITES, AND MYTH

Once you have a successful if not meaningful experience in endurance sports, a part of how you will remember it will depend on how you define it. When you were a kid, sport was often constructed around play. Now, with endurance imputed in the definition of your physical choices, it sure seems like work. What role does the ideal of play versus work take in how we remember the pleasure/effort effect of our sport experience? James (1962), wrestling with how to define an "ideal" in his work toward describing a "significant life" suggested, "an ideal, for instance, must be something intellectually conceived, something of which we are not unconscious, if we 'have it; and it must carry with it that sort of outlook, uplift, and brightness that go with all intellectual facts" (304).

Still, when we drink in the moments that remind us every day how lucky we are as athletes, not so much illuminating the present but exploring the complex interplay between past and future, between work and play, between ideal and idealism, we are apt to swallow those immutably honest moments of athleticism because we know that someday, somehow, we will need that power of ruminative memory. In addition, those memories tend to take on more of an aura of pure chance and creativity than intellectual fact. These are a few of my pure moments:

I remember finishing one of my first Ironman Triathlon World Championship races in Kona and looking down to see that my white shoes were now red. I thought, *Didn't I have white shoes?* Then I remembered it was blood from the blisters. And I remember the Medical Director, Bob Laird, sitting me down, taking off my shoes and cleaning up those blisters, Jesus-like. I remember a local Hawaiian named Curt Tyler walking over and giving me his brand new sandals right off his feet so that I could walk to my hotel over the hot asphalt. Someone told me he was the mayor of the town; just some local *haole* playing a universal earth-deity for the day. I will never forget. It now feels like myth but I know it to be true because I lived it.

I remember not believing it when I was actually in the lead of a major race for the first time, until I slowed down and let the sound of my own breath enter the picture. It became a kind of soundtrack to this movie I was watching; only I was staring in the movie, living two lives at the same time. One was real and one was make believe, but I could not tell the difference at the time until I let all my senses join in the battle and heard the television helicopters following me overhead. I had inherited the mythic simply by swimming, cycling, and running faster than my competitors.

I remember going to the bank and depositing a prize money check for something like $7,500 and thinking that I had lived a full and rewarding year in college for half of that during the 1970s. I told myself not to get used to it. But I think I went out and bought a new guitar that afternoon. It sounded just the same as my old one. I wondered what had changed. Was it was my right to materialize my physical success?

I know many people who occupy themselves with activities they mostly consider unimportant. But observed thoughtfully, they are regular rites of passage. Still, those who consider endurance sport relatively unimportant when compared to family, health, academics, religion, the economy or the environment fail to realize that we have developed *relationships* with all those important elements of society *through* endurance sports. That imputes a degree of import.

When it comes to explaining meaning and motive in endurance sports there are, of course, myriad questions of an ethical nature; particularly within recommendation or pedagogy. Would I suggest, for example, there is more value in seeking an endurance sport support group or by trudging on alone in search of some personal truth? Is it ethically more defensible to follow the lead of groundbreaking athletes in service of their bravery than their coveted style? We remind ourselves that you can purchase an en vogue appearance but that doesn't mean you have style. America's preeminent middle-distance runner of the early 1970s, Steve Prefontaine, ran in baggy T-shirts and dark-colored socks not because they were all the rage. But because they could be purchased inexpensively at secondhand stores.

To ethically question the time-honored quest for youth is to challenge notions of survivorship if not immortality. If an athlete chooses an aerobic sport for its weight management attributes in an effort to remain attractive to a mate, who are we to suggest their motives are any less altruistic than "running for world peace" or "swimming to save the gray whale"? Certainly, the level of cause-association within endurance sports events has reached dizzying levels. A nonprofit association seems almost necessary to attract participants in mass endurance events. But that element may only affect the meaning or motive for the individual if they allow it to do so.

I find cosmetic fitness—the runner who'd rather fit into size four jeans than take home a trophy—refreshing for its candor and the hidden ancillary benefits. And I find the lessons of manufactured myth—when the lessons are clear and cogent—both valuable and entertaining. There was a story bantered around endurance sport circles some years ago that told the tale of a middle-aged man suffering from clinical depression. Apparently, this poor individual attempted suicide-by-running; hoping that he'd suffer a massive and fatal cardiac event while running that would end his life and his depression. Unsuccessful at first, the man continued to run further and further each day. As the tale is told, at the end of one month his mood had improved, he'd lost weight, gained perspective, and gave up his suicidal ideations. And he kept running.

I may have begun this song as the naïve troubadour many years ago, but now, even after the wounds of reentry have healed, I wonder if I had subversively and in sequence convinced myself that it is the endurance game that gives us life; that play comes before player, events before eventuality, and spirit before sport. As endurance athletes, by definition we must go to our borders to find our center. There is meaning in suffering, we tell ourselves, but not in stupidity. These are not unattainable concepts for people who are drawn to a raw and pure form of sport rather than the other minefields of postmodern life; that Halliburton zeitgeist or the new tyranny of the datasphere; Thoreau's "civilization" or the multiplicity of his Walden mindset. Still, you could also live a sedate and vicarious existence and if it is your truth and you are happy, who can argue? One person's championship ring is another's pop-top from an old cola can. Lest we forget, myth is formed in the creation, not the result.[10]

At times, endurance sports participation can seem so distant, so insurmountable, so elusive. But it's not that hard, really. And while it should end in respect, it should also begin there as well—a respect for your dream, your quest, your pleasure in the artful elements, your people, and your memories. You might get there; you might not. As endurance athletes, we cannot resist our motives any more than we can an early morning run when sleeping late would improve our performance. The thrill of filling out a race entry or buying a new pair of athletic shoes is both an asset and our Achilles.

*(Some ideas, concepts, and passages above have been discussed and used in the author's 2015 book, Finding Triathlon: How Endurance Sports Explains Human Behavior. All rights extended.)*

## NOTES

1. What I am suggesting with the "banality of somatics" is that while the body can thrill and teach it can also feel as a tether when the physical life becomes a sought-after and purposeful quest as modern science slowly removes our need to move.

2. Emerson, Carlyle, and Joseph Campbell all approach the notion of heroics and from different but intersecting planes. The reader is advised to compare and contrast how their notions of herodom apply to motives of endurance sport participation.

3. First published in his 1841 collection, *Essays*, Self-Reliance and much of its transcendentalist ideas were appropriated by later writers and athletes including Amby Burfoot, Alan Sillitoe, and John L. Parker.

4. For a period during the first wave of popularity in jogging (1972–1982), the periodical *Runner's World* served readers with ample street philosophy, much of it written by columnist, George Sheehan and editor, Amby Burfoot. Thousands of runners shared their ideas as sacred texts.

5. Thoreau's *Walden or Life in the Woods*, first published in 1854, still stands as de facto bible for those endurance athletes taken to primarily participate outdoors in a natural environment.

6. A similar melding of fashion function, and fitness would finally come to American cycling in the late 1990s. By the 2015, road cycling among the middle and upper classes was so popular that it was labeled "the new golf."

7. Henry Bugbee's 1958 philosophical journal, *The Inward Morning*, provides a pattern for contemplative athletes who chronicle their days' efforts in training logs.

8. John L. Parker's 1978 (republished in 2008) *Once a Runner*, is regarded as the classic exemplar of endurance sport fiction. Almost cultish in popularity among runners, signed original texts have become highly collectible.

9. In 2015, the Ironman Triathlon brand and its properties were sold to a Chinese media and real estate company for a reported $900m. The M-Dot logo tattoo remains a sought-after badge for those desiring a corporate logo as fleshy signifier.

10. Joseph Campbell, in his 1972 book, *Myths to Live By* (Viking Press, NYC), argues that "the function of ritual, as I understand it, is to give form to human life, not in the mere surface arrangement, but in depth" (44). I would argue that our motivation to participate in endurance sports is also catalyzed in a social need for ritual.

# REFERENCES

Atkinson, M. (2008). Triathlon, suffering and exciting significance. *Leisure Studies* 27(2), 165–180.

Bugbee, H. (1999). *The inward morning*. Athens, GA: The University of Georgia Press.

Emerson, R.W. (1981). Circles. In *The portable Emerson*. New York, NY: Penguin Books.

Giddens, A. (1991). *Modernity and self-identity: Self and society in the late modern age*. Stanford, CA: Stanford University Press.

Hochstetler, D. & Hopsicker, P. (2016). Normative concerns for endurance athletes. *Journal of the Philosophy of Sport*, 43(3), 335–349.

James, W. (1962). What makes a life significant? In *Essays on faith and morals*, 285–310. Cleveland, OH: Meridian Books.

Jameson, F. (1998). *The cultural turn: Selected writings on the postmodern 1983–1998*. New York, NY: Verso.

Lasch, C. (1979). *The culture of narcissism: American life in an age of diminishing expectations*. New York, NY: Norton.

Murakami, H. (2008). *What I talk about when I talk about running*. Toronto, ON: Random House.

Parker, J.L. (1990). *Once a runner*. New York, NY: Scribner.

Sheehan, G. (1978). *Running & being: The total experience*. New York, NY: Warner Books.

Sillitoe, A. (1959). *The loneliness of the long-distance runner*. New York, NY: Signet.

Suits, B. (1978). *The grasshopper: Games, life, and utopia*. New York, NY: Broadview Press.

Thoreau, H. (2012). *The portable Thoreau* (J. Cramer, Ed.). New York, NY: Penguin Books.

Williams, W.C. (1951). *The autobiography of William Carlos Williams*. New York, NY: Random House.

# Conclusion

## *Circles of Life: Evaluating Goals and Preparing for the Future*

Douglas Hochstetler

On most mornings, I head out the door for my daily run, in the early morning hours but after a first cup of coffee and quick glance at the local newspaper online. My path varies from day to day but, in general, I head in a southeastern direction—one which provides the most interesting pathways and opportunities. I move slowly during the first half-mile or so and then gradually increase my speed to a sustainable effort. Crossing Cedar Crest Boulevard, I make my way in the direction of J. Birney Crum stadium or, on other days, take a lap through Trexler Park. Regardless of the specific route, my runs are inevitably loops of some variety as I move from the comforts of home, out into the natural surroundings, and then back to home once again.

Over the course of the last four years, my Wednesday morning running routine entails joining a handful of other enthusiasts at the Muhlenberg College track. Each week, after a short warm-up run together, our intrepid group leader details the workout. For example, a sample training session may entail 8 × 400 meters with 400 meters recovery between, followed by 4 × 200 meters with 200-meter recovery. Another week may include a series of 1,000 meter repeats, or various assorted combinations roughly equaling 3 miles of "work." We complete these tasks at our respective speeds, ending the workout together with a slow 1-mile cooldown, circling the track clockwise and finishing our workout in the same place we began.

Ralph Waldo Emerson, although perhaps not a runner or endurance athlete, nonetheless provides a fitting theme for this concluding chapter. In his essay *Circles*, Emerson (1981) goes to great length to describe the various ways circles pervade the natural surroundings. He writes: "The eye is the first circle; the horizon which it forms is the second; and throughout nature this primary picture is repeated without end" (228). Endurance sport participation certainly provides readily apparent examples related to this circular theme. Perhaps most obvious, endurance athletes often compete in events (or complete training sessions) that have one loop, starting and finishing at, or at least nearby, the same place. While point-to-point races and training sessions do occur, they are certainly not the norm. Additionally, the training season itself, like the calendar year, has a rhythm and consistent periods or cycles: from pre-season to in-season to post-season. Or, more specific to each race, a time of building a base, moving toward increasing intensity of workouts, a period of tapering, the event itself, and finally the postrace period before starting another training cycle. Indeed, even the daily workout process has its own circular process—the warm-up, workout, cooldown, recovery—with a similar process on subsequent days.

This circular nature of the endurance athlete's life lends itself to numerous periods of new beginnings, of testing opportunities that may bring about the experiences Dewey emphasized. Endurance sport participation allows us to experience the world differently as compared to a stationary or sedentary position. As Sanders (1995) underscores, "we need to move in loops, out and back again, exploring our home ground, as owls or foxes or indigenous people explore the territory they use for hunting, gathering, mating, and play" (159). If a marathon race goes particularly bad, for example, the runner has opportunities to learn from this experience, or perhaps merely shrug it off, and embark on another marathon-training plan and, perhaps, race. For the cyclist who accomplishes a single day event, a multiday endeavor may provide additional challenges.

Part of Emerson's essay focuses on suffering and the extent to which one might cope with struggle, difficulty, and loss. This was not merely an academic endeavor on his part as Emerson lost his first wife, Ellen, in 1831. "Valor consists in the power of self-recovery," Emerson wrote, "so that a man cannot have his flank turned, cannot be out generalled, but put him where you will, he stands" (233). The endurance sport athlete faces constant possibility of experiencing difficulty through suffering and disappointment, both in the process of training and individual workout sessions and in the competitive testing environment. Upon facing a particularly unsettling setback—failing to qualify for the Boston Marathon, for example—the runner might heed Emerson's advice of "forgetfulness." This short memory of unattained goals then helps drive the athlete toward future training and subsequent aims. Suffering is a constant part of speed workouts and long runs, specific forms of suffering which, the athlete hopes, will lead to faster times and greater distances completed. Becoming acquainted with the harsh environment that is pain enables one to endure this form of experience as a means for growth. John L. Parker (2009), in *Once a Runner,* describes the life, training, and subsequent suffering of a certain miler:

> Quenton Cassidy was not enthusiastically going about the heady business of breaking world records or capturing some coveted prize; such ideas would have been laughable to him in the bland grind of his daily lifestyle. He was merely trying to slip into a lifestyle that he could live with, strenuous but not unendurable by any means, out of which if the corpuscles and the capillaries and the electrolytes were properly aligned in their own mysterious configurations, he might do even better what he had already done quite well. (180)

Despite the intensity of training and the milestones achieved, Cassidy, like other endurance athletes, realized that endurance sport provides unending possibilities and opportunities. As Emerson (1981) puts it, "around every circle another can be drawn; that there is no end in nature, but every end is a beginning" (228). For the endurance athlete, the end of each training cycle, which may culminate in a race day or some other form of testing, presents opportunities for subsequent cycles. Finishing an open water swim, the athlete may evaluate the outcome in light of the training plan, life events, and use this information to develop future training plans and endurance challenges. In the phrasing of Sailors and Cash, they tweak the recipe based on previous experience, adjusting the "ingredients" to improve upon the final product. Another race cycle will provide additional experience and information, an ongoing research study of one. Further, the nature of training plans lend themselves to continual experimentation with training methods, nutritional choices, recovery steps, and so forth.

Future research in this area of American philosophy as it relates to endurance sport depends on both the individual and the broader academic (and athletic) communities. Emerson (1981) described the life we have been given as:

> A self-evolving circle, which, from a ring imperceptibly small, rushes on all sides outwards to new and larger circles, and that without end. The extent to which this generation of circles, wheel without wheel, will go, depends on the force or truth of the individual soul. (230)

Moving forward with this research topic entails moving toward new and larger circles, so to speak, working to understand both the new areas of insight as it relates to endurance sport and the new areas of insight related to American philosophy. Some of these items may involve relatively personal experiences, those that hold significant meaning for the individual athlete but perhaps not for the larger community. Alternatively, other areas of interest and study—hopefully the insights found in this book—encompass a broader scope of potential impact, reaching other endurance sport athletes and/or other scholars focused on American philosophy. That said, the chapters contained in this work do not represent the totality of endurance sport perspectives related to American philosophy. For example, the perspectives of the previous chapters are primarily North American, male, and individuals for whom endurance sport is a significant identity marker. We fully recognize this scope and leave it to other writers to draw from their own lens of experience and background.

Continuing to train and experience life through the lens of an endurance athlete provides ongoing opportunities for growth. This particular endurance sport angle of vision holds endless possibilities for not only physiological development but related to academic insights as well. To the attentive individual, the backdrop of running, cycling, or swimming provides a wealth of experiences that may prove fruitful for personal and academic growth. For example, Fry writes about the notions of will and belief, in the context of endurance sport. He writes not only from and through his academic lens of philosophy and religious studies, but also as an endurance athlete himself. Fry understands the experiential depth of long-distance training, what it feels like to hit the proverbial "wall" and to summon the will, somehow, to keep going.

Throughout this book, the focus has been on the transactional relationship between endurance sport and American philosophy. Each chapter has included a different point of emphasis and corresponding different angle of vision. At this point, my aim is to reflect on the previous chapters to focus on three specific questions. First, what have we learned about endurance sport? Second, what have we learned about American philosophy? Finally, what questions remain that might provide fertile ground for future research? I will explore these questions in turn, keeping in mind that the nature of endurance sport and American philosophy function in tandem; to describe them separately is not only difficult but also not entirely accurate.

In terms of endurance sport, it is possible to glean from the insights raised by the authors, insights earned through the collective years of experience dedicated to various forms of endurance sport, in combination with an academically inclined angle of vision. Illundain et al, for example, point out the nuanced and transactional relationship between the endurance sport athlete and the environment, and in particular their description of the open water swimmer. As endurance athletes gradually become immersed in their respective practice, the dualistic relationship between athlete and nature (conceptualized broadly) collapses. The swimmer takes on the characteristics of the water. The biker, as Kretchmar illustrates, takes on qualities of the bike. In this manner, the bike becomes an extension of the biker, not a tool as much as an additional appendage.

In addition to the transactional nature of endurance sport athletes and the environment, as any endurance sport athlete recognizes, the experience of pushing oneself in an informal training session or competitive race environment entails a certain degree of suffering. This situation brings about an opportunity to both endure and potentially learn from this quality of being.

Fry, for example, addresses the aspect of suffering in endurance sport, asking how it is possible to face and conquer such pain and distress. He points us toward the American philosophical tradition, most notably to William James, to help understand the place of the will, of belief, and of the self with respect to the impact on endurance sport athletes and their situations. The nature of the suffering is important too in that these athletes chose to endure a certain type of very specific pain, one predicated on staying physically active for an extended period of time.

As the endurance sport athletes become more committed to the practice community, these individuals may be tempted to pursue their activity in potentially damaging or unhealthy ways. Tinley provides illustration here, with his hopes to run a quick five-miler while his wife is in labor. Other current examples of unhealthy or damaging behaviors arise in the form of cheating, performance enhancement drug use, or too much time spent apart from family and loved ones. Here American philosophy, in particular Dewey (as pointed out by Illundain), may provide a pathway forward. When properly understood, the notion of Deweyan habits may operate in a way which helps endurance sport athletes maintain a "suppleness of character." Here, habits are not actions which lead to "inflexibility, uncreative doggedness" but rather toward a "Deweyan flexibility habit and dynamic deliberation" (Illundain, et al.).

Finally, and perhaps most importantly, many of the contributors intimate, and some state explicitly, the potential for endurance sport to function in a way which promotes good lives in an Aristotelian, human flourishing sort of way. Anderson, for example, highlights the importance of running for its potential in helping individuals carve out opportunities for personal reflection and musement. In the same manner in which Thoreau wrote about his experience at Walden Pond, endurance sport may, for some, serve as a human practice conducive to a life well lived. The point here is not that everyone take up running, cycling, swimming, or other endurance sport pursuits per se, but rather that the unique experiential aspects of these activities may be beneficial in ways which go well beyond merely physiological qualities—ways which enhance both individual lives and the broader surroundings in meaningful ways.

In the same manner of gleaning insights regarding endurance sport, this book has also distilled important information and ideas regarding American philosophy. Some of these insights have come about in a way reminiscent of Henry Bugbee (1999) describing his graduate school philosophy experience: "I studied philosophy in the classroom and at a desk, but my philosophy took shape mainly on foot. It was truly peripatetic, engendered not merely while walking, but *through* walking that was essentially a *meditation of the place*" (139). I summarize here not in an exhaustive manner, but in ways illustrative of how reflection on endurance sport, and *through* endurance sport, may help provide insights related to American philosophy.

Illundain and colleagues help unpack the notions of situated and enacted stances, an approach to cognition which recognizes the transactional nature of interaction between humanity (and other organisms) and the environment. Further, they unpack these concepts in concert with Dewey's holistic view of humanity, and find endurance sport especially enlightening in this regard. As swimmer Lynn Cox navigates her way through open waters, she encounters a vast array of experiential qualities—water temperature and salinity, size and nature of waves, wind direction and speed, marine animals—coupled with her past experiences as a swimmer in similar and dissimilar conditions. Cox "actively and dynamically adapts" to the conditions but in a corresponding manner "the water itself 'responds' differently to her varying stroke speeds, movement patterns, and techniques." Kretchmar, too, identifies the transactional relationship between the biker and the bike. He writes, "my mountain bike is not just a metal object in the garage; she has invaded my person."

In a similar manner, Illundain and colleagues explore Dewey's concept of habits. They explain that rather than using the term habit to connote stasis or mere repetition, Dewey frames the term to encompass ideas of dynamism and continual processes. Thus habits, in this Deweyan sense, engender a flexible stance and are situated within specific contexts. In this way, skilled habits (the term Illundain and colleagues use) "foster creative spaces, for we need to improvise, adapt, and deliberate to meet challenges." Again, runners, cyclists, swimmers, and other endurance athletes provide an embodied model of skilled habits. Offshore sailors, for example, refine their skills in the context of their ocean-specific environment, constantly adapting their movements and decisions based on a fluid interaction with their surroundings. Even ultraendurance feats such as Reinhold Messner crossing Antarctica on foot, perhaps viewed as the epitome of repetitive acts, demonstrate the transactional relationship between the individual and the environment, with ongoing opportunities for growth.

Further, Hopsicker examines the idea of "representative men" put forth by Emerson, the idea that a few exemplary individuals in society may provide guidance in terms of the notion of genius. These people—identified by Emerson as Plato, Swedenborg, Montaigne, Shakespeare, Napoleon, and Goethe—personified qualities of intellectual and/or creative brilliance, living in a manner quite different as compared with the average citizen. Here, endurance sport helps bring evidence to the role of not only individual narratives but collective ones as well. It is not difficult to think of sporting genius, or "representative athletes," in a similar manner, especially when it comes to sports that are more traditional. Those who follow golf may think of Jordan Spieth in this manner, while others with a passion for tennis may look up to Serena Williams. Rather than merely serving as individuals who embody sporting genius, however, Hopsicker contends that endurance athletes may help explain Emerson's representative men in the sense of an endurance community. Since runners and cyclists and swimmers come in contact with a broad swath of humanity and set an exemplary lifestyle example with regard to human movement, these individuals may help encourage sedentary folks to take part in the challenge and pursuit of endurance sport.

Both Fry and Kretchmar identify the nature of uncertainty—a key concept for James and other pragmatists—and the extent to which endurance sport athletes exemplify commitment in the face of constant uncertainty. For William James, acting in situations that are tenuous, where the impending outcome is not clear, necessitates a certain degree of faith. This faith is buttressed by the notion of genuine options, that is if the available possibilities are "live," "forced," and "momentous." James even uses movement-oriented narratives such as climbing the Alps to demonstrate how a degree of faith is required (such as in needing to take a literal leap of faith) in order to survive a dangerous, mountain-climbing ordeal. Endurance athletes provide vivid representations of this faith-inspired quality, summoning up the determination in self to accomplish seemingly insurmountable tasks. William Greer, the Boston Marathon runner to whom Fry refers, appears unable to finish the race without walking, but somehow manages to keep going and run across the finish line. Kretchmar points toward James' notion of significance as a means to think more carefully about the value of uncertainty. On reflection of his time at Chautauqua Lake, James (1962) realized he missed the precipitousness of daily life. "Sweat and effort," he wrote, "human nature strained to its uttermost and on the rack, yet getting through alive, and then turning its back on its success to pursue another more rare still—this is the sort of thing the presence of which inspires us" (290). Endurance sport activities then, with the constant presence of uncertainty, help partially explain and exemplify these philosophical concepts of faith, belief, and significance. Embarking on an ultraendurance test provides very little in the form of certainty—there are so many things that could possibly go wrong. Yet, the very nature of this decision, and the faith upon which it rests, results in the possibility that the individual may experience life in extremis, the very significance of which James spoke.

Elcombe, through his focus on aesthetics, brings forward the Deweyan ideas of human doing and undergoing. Concerning the former, Dewey praises those qualities of action that make a coordinated and impactful difference in one's context. Doing, in this sense, entails human energy pointed toward a particular end, one meaningful and significant. James, too, emphasized the importance of a certain strenuousness, of working to overcome hardship in the pursuit of excellence. Alongside human doing exists the quality of undergoing, understood as a receptive sense of suffering, putting up with, enduring, and making it through. Taken together, these notions of doing and undergoing with respect to endurance sport help to explain the human fascination with sport, and in particular with activities such as endurance sport participation. Pursuits such as bike racing appeal to both the participant and spectator in large measure because of this particular form of doing—of riding up incredibly steep mountain passes, and screaming down the other side at breakneck speed; of riding for countless miles in all types of weather, risking injury daily in the process.

Moreover, endurance sport athletes help illustrate, through the course of personal and collective narratives, the place of aesthetics and meaning as part of human flourishing. Tinley provides a first-person example here, as he works to identify personal meaning in the context of his triathlete existence. With elite Ironman experience, Tinley recognizes the extent to which endurance sport excellence may coexist with and even exemplify human flourishing. He also realizes the personal toll required of endurance athletes who become hooked, so to speak, and that this toll may affect the lives of significant others. In a different manner, Anderson speaks to the way in which endurance sport may lead to another form of human flourishing—of living life philosophically. Rather than running, cycling, or swimming with hopes of achieving international renown or even personal best times and/or distances, perhaps it is possible to move for long periods of time, in part, because of the space it provides for reflective thought. It is in this manner, Anderson contends, that endurance sport may function as an opportunity for musement, which may potentially lead toward amelioration of both personal and societal levels.

Finally, in the same manner in which endurance sport athletes may encourage others to move, and to make a broader impact on their surroundings, American philosophy as an academic discipline, and American philosophers in general, has the potential to speak to the broader culture in impactful ways. Contrary to the all-too-familiar role of philosophy in the United States at least, American philosophy indeed holds the potential for relevance and impact for modern society. Many of the American philosophical themes remain credible for a twenty-first-century context. In fact, I would argue that in the same way American philosophers (and Americans in general) benefit from reading texts from other cultures and philosophical themes, others around the world similarly stand to benefit from reading and thinking about the world from the American philosophical angle of vision.

To conclude this chapter and this work, it is fitting to think about ways in which the preceding chapters point us toward potential questions, ones that may be fitting for a classroom setting, some for potential research agendas, and others for personal thought and exploration. In the spirit of American philosophy and endurance sport, life is constantly in flux, with many challenges and opportunities on the horizon. In Emerson's words, we may realize these qualities if we just lift our eyes. The following questions represent a starting point and should not be considered an exhaustive list. Others may encounter questions that resonate with them. That said, the following questions represent a start and are important.

Onwards to the potential questions then. First, Hopsicker raises the notion of impact of endurance sport for the broader contemporary society. It is one thing to experience the gamut of available qualia through running, swimming, or biking. With knowledge that so many people in Western culture (in the United States especially) lead sedentary lives, it seems unjust to not be concerned with this pocket of humanity. In more practical terms, how might endurance sport athletes both encourage and support the non-mover? Surely, there are both practical and theoretical avenues available. At a minimum, those readers who count themselves as endurance sport enthusiasts might think of their own narrative concerning endurance sport. To what extent did other people influence their decision to become an endurance athlete? What was that relationship like? How, and for what reasons, did they start to train and, possibly, compete? To what extent, and in what manner, has this brought about significance or meaning? These questions are ripe for additional reflection and research.

Second, Elcombe, channeling Dewey, prompts us to think about the place of aesthetics in endurance sport as well as the broader culture. The guiding question here is how we might structure our lives such to live in a more artful manner. What would that look like and how might we encourage others to join in this pursuit of an aesthetically pleasing life? American philosophers, like Thoreau, took this question very seriously. For Thoreau, addressing this question led to his intentional two-year experiment living beside Walden Pond. During this time Thoreau dedicated himself to living in an attentive and artful manner, focused on "living deliberately" and writing about this experience for readers to understand. For endurance sport athletes, living artfully may not necessarily entail moving to the woods for an extended time—although perhaps this could be beneficial—but rather how best to structure one's training, racing, and broader aspects of life such to live in this artful manner, deliberate and attentive and full.

Third, stories of specific individual endurance athletes, like Floyd Landis, may provide additional fodder for continued research in this area of endurance sport related to American philosophy. What other athlete narratives might serve as "ideal muse" for our continued pursuit? This might be in the form of exemplary feats of competition-related excellence (e.g., setting a new record, finishing a particularly grueling race) or as part of an extended training program or individual narrative (e.g., individuals harmed in the Boston Marathon bombing who trained for and ran subsequent races, or cyclists who remained resilient in their training despite personal tragedy). Additionally, these stories may involve personal encounters—researchers who think and write about their own experiences with endurance sport. It may also involve thinking and writing about others, both those in the elite category of endurance sport participation and those at other levels of commitment.

Fourth, how do other philosophical traditions relate to both American philosophy and endurance sport? Welters helps us understand the potential for this kind of pursuit, pointing toward the relationship between continental thought and American philosophy, but many other possibilities are likely. American philosophers such as Thoreau were familiar with and read widely from other wisdom traditions—Protestant Christianity, Eastern philosophy, Native American writing, and so forth. As Thoreau spent time at Walden, for example, he continually worked toward developing his own philosophical style and positions. He did this by immersing himself in his surroundings, paying close attention to the pond, the woods, the animals, and other natural surroundings, and by drawing from his own thought process buttressed by his extensive reading. His writing provides evidence of this attention to nature in constant dialogue of sorts with connections to his personal life, to broader societal issues, and often referencing terms or ideas from his wealth of knowledge and reading.

Fifth, Tinley provides a superlative example of an ongoing questioning spirit within the context of personal narrative. For those who identify as enthusiasts, in terms of both endurance sport and philosophy, a lifelong pursuit of endurance sport provides a rich context for like-minded individuals seeking and asking questions. Even though Tinley has trained and competed in triathlon-related activities for decades, he continues to ask questions related to purpose. His reasons for participating in endurance sport early in his career are different from his reasons for participating now. Nonetheless, he continues to think about the meaning of these pursuits, both for himself and for the broader triathlon and endurance sport community. For those whose daily pursuits involve running, cycling, and swimming, the commitment toward these activities and the kind of lives produced engender an ongoing possibility for questioning. This questioning spirit might relate to overall purpose, or it might encompass other areas such as ethics, aesthetics, axiology, or other philosophical areas of thought.

Finally, as Anderson notes, endurance sport practices such as running can be helpful in ameliorating future problems. Here, I mean that time spent moving enables a sort of musing that may be fruitful on many fronts—both personal and broader to the societal level. This requires an attentiveness on the part of the participant for sure, a stance toward endurance sport wherein the activity is not pursued solely, or even primarily, for health-related goals. For those who run, bike, swim—those who are serious about these activities, and identify as runners, bikers, or swimmers—and think about these pursuits at length, their musings are noteworthy and we should, in general and as a culture, listen to these stories and insights. As Anderson argues for "a genuine conversation among our philosophical outlooks, a conversation in which we listen closely not only to each other's arguments, but also to the stories we tell *about* and *from* the perspectives of our experiential homes" (7). As we seek philosophical insights with hopes of ameliorating some of our current challenges, Anderson reminds us to listen not only to cogent philosophical points, but also to those points grounded in personal experience. In this way, endurance sport pursuits count in the radical empiricism of William James, because these experiences (and our stories) tell others not only about the richness of endurance sport, but also about the angle of vision from which we face the world. In this way the perspective of endurance athletes adds to the broader philosophical tradition, enriching the overall conversation that is linked through James and Thoreau, Dewey and Rorty.

Through the course of this book, we have examined many important areas of thought related to both endurance sport and American philosophy. As authors, our task has involved thinking carefully about both areas of study and how each area intersects with and relates to the other, or perhaps more accurately, the transactional nature of endurance sport and American philosophy. Despite our best attempts of seeking clarity and guiding the reader in this effort, we also acknowledge, faithful to our pragmatic spirit, that our attempts will not produce any final clarity. We invite others, perhaps from different perspectives and backgrounds, to take up this topic of endurance sport and American philosophy also. Borrowing from Emerson (1981) here, "Thus there is no sleep, no pause, no preservation, but all things renew, germinate and spring" (238). For the writers and I, this is our best understanding of the topics right now. In time, with more miles training and, perhaps, competitive testing experiences under our belt, with other books and articles read, we may approach the same questions differently, or develop additional questions to pursue. To this end, I want to close with a quote from Emerson (1981):

> The one thing which we seek with insatiable desire is to forget ourselves, to be surprised out of our propriety, to lose our sempiternal memory and to do something without knowing how or why; in short to draw a new circle. Nothing great was ever achieved without enthusiasm. (240)

In that spirit, I have a new running route I want to explore.

## REFERENCES

Bugbee, H. (1999). *The inward morning.* Athens, GA: The University of Georgia Press.
Emerson, R. (1981). Circles. In *The portable Emerson.* New York, NY: Penguin Books, pp. 228–240.
James, W. (1962). *Essays on faith and morals.* Cleveland, OH: Meridian Books.
Parker, J.L. (2009). *Once a runner.* New York, NY: Scribner Publishing.
Sanders, S. (1995). *Writing from the center.* Bloomington, IN: Indiana University Press.

# Index

abduction, 2–3
aesthetics, 31–48, 165–67
American philosophy, xiii–xxv, 32, 35, 144, 161–69
analytic philosophy, 14, 57
asceticism, 17–28

belonging, xxix
body-mind, 99–120

cash value, 1, 21, 81
certainty, xviii, 41, 46, 165
commitment, xiii, xxvi–xxxi, 23, 32–34, 50, 65, 72–73, 99, 118, 127, 130, 165, 168
community, xiii, xvii, xix–xx, xxii, xxvi, xxviii–xxix, 7, 34, 53, 63, 65, 71–74, 83, 86, 89, 117–19, 151, 161, 163, 165, 168
computational and representational stance (CRS), 99–118
constitutive rules, 51
continental philosophy, 11, 14

doing and undergoing, 32, 41–46, 165–66
dualism, 100–101, 111

embodied cognition, 99

endurance athlete, xvii, xix, xxii–xxv, xxvii, 24–25, 36–40, 43–44, 62–64, 74, 79, 117, 126–27, 129–30, 132–33, 135, 138, 143–45, 148, 150, 152, 155–56, 159–62, 164–69
ethics, xiv, xxi, 24–25, 42–43, 168
experiential, xx, xxiv, xxvii, xxxi, 2–4, 7–8, 32, 35, 42, 97, 102, 112, 119, 126, 143, 162–64, 169

fair play, 14, 108
faith, 82, 127–31, 165
fallibilism, xxvii, 86
flow, 15, 115, 131–32
formalists, 14
foundationalism, 84–85
free will, 132–38

games, 13–18, 24, 32, 44, 51–54, 107, 149
genius, 61–74
genuine option, 128–30, 165
good life, xiii, 9, 22, 25

habits, 2–3, 8–9, 20–21, 103–7, 113–17, 163–64
human flourishing (eudaimonia), 12, 24

identity, xv, xxiii–xxv, 24, 126, 146–47, 162

## Index

imaginative phronesis (IP), 107–8, 120
immersion, xxix, 15, 120
inner terrain, 6–7
internal goods, 63–65
interpretivists, 14
intimacy, xxviii–xxix

lusory attitude, 15

meditation, 3–8, 58, 134, 138, 163
meliorism, xvii, xxvii, xxix–xxx, 12, 58
musement, 2–9, 163, 166

pain, xxiii–xxiv, 1, 41, 45, 112, 115–17, 126, 137, 143, 145–48, 151, 160, 163
phenomenological, 2, 62, 116, 150
philosophy of sport, xx, 14–15
phronesis, 107–8, 120
play, 4–5, 13–15, 18, 50, 52–54, 144, 153–55
pluralism, xvii
practice, xiii, xx, xxiii, xxviii, 2–9, 11–12, 17–23, 27, 41–43, 46, 61, 63–69, 74, 91, 93–95, 103–4, 108, 110, 113–20, 162–63, 168
pragmatism, xiv, xvii, 12, 21, 23, 28, 36, 41, 46, 79–91, 152
precipitousness, xx, xxx, 53, 69, 165
progress, xxvi–xxvii, 3, 34, 54–55, 58, 72

radical empiricism, xvii, 80, 169
radical enactivism, 103
receptivity, 6, 8
reflection, xiv, xxii, 3, 6, 8, 95, 113, 117, 135, 164–65
relativism, 85, 91

repetitive practice (askesis), 11, 17–18, 27–28
risk, xx, xxvii, xxx, 38, 43, 45, 89, 102, 104, 107–9, 112–13, 119, 144–46, 149, 166

self, xxiii, xxviii–xxix, 8–9, 21–28, 41, 49–50, 64–67, 115–17, 126–38, 153, 163, 165
significance, xiii, xvii, xix, xxxi, 41, 50, 52, 55–59, 110, 114, 129, 165, 167
simplicity, xiv–xv, 37, 62
situated and enactive account (SEA), 100
skilled habit (SH), 108, 120
social cognition, 99, 114
solitude, xiv, xx, xxii, 70
sport philosophy, xxi, 13
strenuous life, 25, 36, 40, 98, 126
suffering, xiii, xxiii, 1, 6, 23, 28, 32, 39–41, 112, 126, 151, 155, 160, 162–63, 166

techne, 5
transactional, 85, 104–5, 115–16, 120, 162, 164, 169
transcendentalism, xv–xvi, 23
transcendentalists, xxiv, 64
truth, xix, xxix, 11, 14–16, 19–21, 27, 41, 43, 67–68, 79–95, 99, 117, 128, 154–55, 161

virtue ethics, 24–25

wildness, 71
wisdom, xx–xxi, xxvii, 2–3, 9, 16, 24–25, 64, 75, 120, 130, 168
working utopians, xix, xxvii

# Contributor Biographies

**Douglas Anderson** studies the history of philosophy and American philosophy, and is interested in philosophy's relationship to other dimensions of culture. Therefore, his work covers a range of fields from philosophy of science and religion to philosophy of sport, music, and education. Authors of particular interest to him at present include Thoreau, bell hooks, Gloria Anzaldúa, Plato, and Henry Bugbee. His traditional work in American Philosophy focuses on Charles Peirce and the history of pragmatism.

**Kaarina Beam** is Assistant Professor of Philosophy at Linfield College (United States), where she has been engaged in the scholarship of teaching since 1999 and served as chair of the philosophy department for more than ten years. She specializes in American philosophies, value theory, and the philosophy of education. Her areas of research coalesce around her interest in the enculturation of selves through institutionalized systems. Her current research is focused on the habits of mind and character that enable a civic-centered education to function as the cornerstone of a fiduciary democracy.

**Amby Burfoot** won the 1968 Boston Marathon, served as Runner's World editor in chief for nearly two decades, and finished the 2018 Boston Marathon on the 50th anniversary of his victory. He has run 110,000 lifetime miles, and his most recent book is titled *Run Forever*.

**Cody D. Cash**, PhD, is an instructor in the Philosophy Department at Missouri State University. His latest work has focused on embodied cognition. Cody is a recent convert to competitive running after decades of soccer; he has completed one marathon, with more on the horizon.

**Tim Elcombe**, an Associate Professor in Kinesiology and Physical Education at Wilfrid Laurier University in Waterloo, Ontario, Canada, received his PhD from Penn State University. His research focuses on addressing ethical issues emerging in sporting contexts, exploring intersections between sport and culture, and examining uses of sport as a sociopolitical tool. Publishing in journals including the *International Journal of the History of Sport*, the *Journal of the Philosophy of Sport*, the *Journal of Canadian Studies*, and the *SAIS Review of International Affairs*, he was awarded the British Philosophy of Sport Association's Developing Researcher Award in 2010.

**Jeffrey Fry** is an Associate Professor in the Department of Philosophy and Religious Studies at Ball State University. He serves on the editorial boards of the *Journal of the Philosophy of Sport* and *Sport, Ethics and Philosophy*. He has also served as a member at large on the executive council of the International Association for the Philosophy of Sport. His interests include the philosophy of sport, ethics, the philosophy of mind, neurophilosophy, the philosophy of religion, and the intersection of these disciplines.

**Shaun Gallagher** is the Lillian and Morrie Moss Chair of Excellence in Philosophy at the University of Memphis (2011–present). He holds a secondary appointment as Professorial Fellow on the Faculty of Law, Humanities and the Arts, at the University of Wollongong (Australia). From 2007 to 2015, he held a secondary appointment as Research Professor of Philosophy and Cognitive Science at the University of Hertfordshire (UK). He is Honorary Professor of Philosophy at the University of Durham (UK), and Honorary Professor of Health Sciences at the University of Tromsø in Norway. He is the recipient of the Humboldt Foundation's first Anneliese Maier Research Award (2012–2017). Among his many acclaimed books are *Phenomenology* (Palgrave, 2012), *The Phenomenological Mind*, 2nd edition, with Dan Zahavi (Routledge, 2012), and *How the Body Shapes the Mind* (Oxford University Press, 2005). He is also a founding editor, and continues as a co-editor-in-chief of the journal *Phenomenology and the Cognitive Sciences*. His areas of research include phenomenology and the cognitive sciences, especially topics related to embodiment, self, agency, and intersubjectivity.

**Douglas Hochstetler** is interested in philosophical issues related to sport and physical activity, with an emphasis on American philosophy as it relates to running and other endurance sport pursuits. As Professor of Kinesiology, Hochstetler currently serves as Director of Academic Affairs at Penn State University, Lehigh Valley. He is past Editor of *Quest* (the official journal of the National Association for Kinesiology in Higher Education) and has served as guest reviewer for both *Kinesiology Review* and *Sport, Ethics and*

Philosophy. A former college team-sport athlete, his endurance sport experiences include two cycling trips across the United States, numerous marathons and half-marathons.

**Peter M. Hopsicker** serves as Professor of Kinesiology at Penn State Altoona. He has authored and coauthored several papers examining endurance sport through a pragmatic, experiential lens. Additionally, Dr. Hopsicker often uses the works of Michael Polanyi to investigate cognition in motor behavior—the differences between "knowing how" (practical knowledge) and "knowing that" (prepositional knowledge)—and also investigates the interplay of sport and spirituality. Finally, he is very active within the subdiscipline contributing several analyses of the current state and future promise of sport philosophy. Dr. Hopsicker's essays can be found in the *Journal of the Philosophy of Sport*; *Sport, Ethics and Philosophy*; the *International Journal of Physical Education*; the *Journal of Disability and Religion*; *Quest*; and *Kinesiology Review*.

**Daniel D. Hutto** is Professor of Philosophical Psychology at the University of Wollongong (Australia) and the University of Hertfordshire (UK). Currently a Member of the Australian Research Council (ARC) College of Experts, he was a Chief coinvestigator for the ARC "Embodied Virtues and Expertise" project (2010–2013) and a node leader in the Marie Curie Action "Towards an Embodied Science of Intersubjectivity" Initial training network (2011–2015). Among his recent works are *Radicalizing Enactivism* (MIT, 2013), a Choice Outstanding Academic Title 2013, and *Folk Psychological Narratives* (MIT, 2008). His recent research focuses primarily on issues in philosophy of mind, psychology, and cognitive science.

**Jesús Ilundáin-Agurruza** is Professor and Chair of the Philosophy Department at Linfield College (USA). There, he received the 2011–2012 Samuel H. Graf Faculty Achievement Award and was 2008–2009 Allen & Pat Kelley Faculty Scholar. In 2013–2015, he served as president of the International Association for the Philosophy of Sport (IAPS). He is a former Fellow at the Institute for Philosophy in the Public Life (2010). His most recent publication is *Holism and the Cultivation of Excellence in Sports and Performance: Skillful Striving* (Routledge, 2016). His philosophical interests range from sport philosophy and value theory to the philosophy of mind, extending into East Asian Philosophy (especially Japanese). An avid cyclist, swimmer, and budding free diver, he also enjoys a good sparring bout with his longsword.

**Scott Kretchmar** is Professor of Exercise and Sport Science at Penn State University. He is a founding member of the International Association for the

Philosophy of Sport and served as its President. He has been editor of the *Journal of the Philosophy of Sport*, is a Fellow in the American Academy of Kinesiology and Physical Education, and has authored a popular text in the philosophy of sport. He has published over sixty refereed articles and more than thirty book chapters on such topics as ethics, the nature of sport, and the operation of human intelligence in physical activity. He was named Alliance Scholar for AAHPERD in 1996, received the Distinguished Scholar Award from NAPEHE in 1997, was honored as Distinguished Scholar for the International Association for the Philosophy of Sport in 1998 and again in 2006, and was named the Charles H. McCloy Research Lecturer by the NASPE Research Consortium in 2012. Kretchmar served as Chair of the Department of Kinesiology at Penn State on two occasions, has been President of the University Faculty Senate, and served as the Faculty Athletics Representative to the NCAA from 2001 to 2010. He was the founding editor of the *Journal of Intercollegiate Sport* and served four years as Chairman of the Board for the NCAA Scholarly Colloquium.

**Pam R. Sailors**, PhD, is a professor in the Philosophy Department and Associate Dean of the College of Humanities and Public Affairs at Missouri State University. Her recent work in philosophy of sport has addressed running, roller derby, gender, American football, and issues of equity. Pam is a competitive runner who has completed more than three dozen half marathons and forty full marathons.

**Scott Tinley**, a seventh generation southern Californian, has been a freelance writer and university lecturer longer than he was a professional athlete. He has published five volumes of nonfiction, a collection of short fiction and numerous texts in literary journals. Tinley holds a PhD in Cultural Studies from Claremont Graduate University, an MA in Interdisciplinary Studies, and an MFA in Fiction. Much of his research surrounds new approaches to considering athletes in retirement and transition. He teaches sport humanities courses at SDSU and CSUSM. A former paramedic and sailing instructor Tinley's favorite job is still working as a seasonal lifeguard on the beaches of Del Mar, California where he lives with his wife and two grown children. He rarely thinks about his twenty years racing the IRONMAN Triathlon in Hawaii.

**Ron Welters** is with the Institute for Science, Innovation and Society of Radboud University in The Netherlands. In 2018, he finished his PhD thesis entitled "Towards a Sustainable Philosophy of Endurance Sport—Cycling for Life." He is an ardent long-distance cyclist and runner.

www.ingramcontent.com/pod-product-compliance
Lightning Source LLC
Chambersburg PA
CBHW050905300426
44111CB00010B/1390